Lightning at the Gate

Lightning at the Gate

A Visionary Journey of Healing

◇

Jeanne Achterberg

SHAMBHALA

BOSTON & LONDON

2002

To the medicine men who gave so generously of their time and love;
and to the girlfriends, medicine women all, who were ever there

SHAMBHALA PUBLICATIONS, INC.
HORTICULTURAL HALL
300 MASSACHUSETTS AVENUE
BOSTON, MASSACHUSETTS 02115
www.shambhala.com

9 8 7 6 5 4 3 2 1

FIRST EDITION
Printed in the United States of America

⊗ This edition is printed on acid-free paper that meets the
American National Standards Institute z39.48 Standard.
Distributed in the United States by Random House, Inc.,
and in Canada by Random House of Canada Ltd

LIBRARY OF CONGRESS CATALOGING-IN-PUBLICATION DATA
Achterberg, Jeanne.
Lightning at the gate: a visionary journey of healing/Jeanne Achterberg.
p.   cm.
Includes bibliographical references.
ISBN 1-57062-858-0
1. Achterberg, Jeanne—Health.   2. Eye—Cancer—Patients—United
States—Biography.   3. Melanoma—Patients—United
States—Biography.   4. Eye—Cancer—Alternative treatment.
5. Melanoma—Alternative treatment.   I. Title.
RC280.E9 A25 2002
362.1′9699484′092—dc21
[B]   2001042985

Contents

—◇—

Acknowledgments   ix

Prologue   3

Epiphany: Kosovo   12

Homecoming   18

Vision Quest   20

Business as Usual, More or Less   25

Initiation   27

Medical Mystery and Maybe
the Black Widow   31

Dark Flight   35

Grim Reaper Diagnosis   44

Demon Diagnoses   51

Eagles Everywhere   59

Snowballing Support   62

The Big Hand   67

The Medicine Dance Begins   76

What I Need Now   82

Turnaround Time   84

Kill-or-Cure Routine   89

Mistletoe and Dreams   94

Shamanic Healing   102

Girl Talk   110

Detective Work   112

England: A Healing Pilgrimage   117

Ceilidh   124

Days of Reckoning   133

Dark Weeks   135

Germany: Same Time, Next Year   150

The Event   156

Thanksgiving and Transcendence   165

Saint Lucy's Days   173

Young Things   177

Life Returns   179

CONTENTS

Meditation Medicine   185

Matters of a Religious Nature   189

Answered Prayers   192

Valentine   198

Dreamer   202

Unfinished Business   204

And More Dream Helpers   208

Relationship Ruminations   212

What Is Real?   219

Old Bones   222

Birthday   228

Twilight Zone   233

Healing Island   235

Fire in the Mountain   238

Surgery   242

Psyche's Challenges   246

Epilogue   250

RESOURCES   255

Acknowledgments

THIS BOOK ITSELF is a narrative of acknowledgments, a tribute to caring that knows no limits. This story is a tapestry of healing and medical history in the making. Although I have used some fictitious names for privacy, the people behind those names still need to know of my appreciation.

My gratitude is expressed to all those who prayed for me in circles of many spiritual persuasions, whose names I will never know. The E-mails, cards, gifts, songs, and telephone calls from colleagues, students, and friends were a lifeline. Each one came at the perfect moment. I learned from you to feel the tangible effects of prayer; it opened my heart and healed my body.

Other mystics and healers came into my life after the major text was written: Grandfather Raven magically appeared one morning while I was in Mexico to tell me he had been praying for me all night and to remind me I was a survivor and an angel. David Cumes, a physician trained in African shamanism, threw the bones and divined my past, present, and future, giving me ceremonies to reestablish harmony for my health and for my children. Maria, a Greek spiritualist living in Germany, diagnosed the nature of my health, the conditions of my living environment, gave advice on protection, and she and her partner, Peter Lutz, prayed daily for a month. Lanakila Brandt, a *kahuna pule* (a medicine person who uses prayer and spirit for healing), brought this portion of the healing journey full circle with days of songs and chants from the most loving healing tradition on the planet.

My family deserves special acknowledgment: the time has been tumultuous for all of us. We grew into an appreciation of the fact that blood runs very thick indeed. There is an old saying, "My barn has burned down, and now I can see the moon." My barn burned, and now I see my family.

Emily Hilburn Sell, my editor, and Stephanie Tade, my literary agent, are also Medicine Women. They trusted that I would have a book worthy of interest at a time when I was only feebly scratching notes whose direction was uncertain. Maybe an agility with words makes a writer, but so does this kind of unfailing trust.

Lightning at the Gate

If I were to wish for anything,
I should not wish for wealth and power,
but for the passionate sense of the potential,
an eye which, ever young and ardent,
sees the possible.

—SØREN KIERKEGAARD

Prologue

{January 23, 2000}

THIS IS A STORY that does not yet have an ending. I can't say for certain where or when it begins. It is about a time outside of time, a Calypso time when I was captured by the Fates and, like Odysseus, forced to wander the unseen worlds.

Writing to save your life, to give meaning and purpose to tragedy and crisis and mysteries you may never understand, is the most difficult writing on the face of the earth. When you write about life, you have to revisit it, taste and smell it again, analyze it, put it in context. How did Henry Miller, Anaïs Nin, Simone de Beauvoir, Jean-Paul Sartre, Virginia Woolf, and the great biographers and novelists who were really writing about their lives and from their experience, do just that, so often and for so long? Straddling the worlds between what is happening and what is being written is like wearing a boot on one foot and a slipper on the other and trying to waltz. But then, they were writing about politics or philosophy or fucking, and I'm writing about how to stay alive. Maybe that is why this seems such a monumental challenge.

I used to get seriously vexed while reading women's journals from the Wild West when they just recorded events and not their dreams, feelings, or juicy details of their interior lives. As in "Today we buried two of our three children," or "We reached our destination on the prairie and built the sod hut." This was life at the edge. Now I get it. Some days it's all you can do merely to get down the bare-bones facts of what just happened, even when you're trying to keep careful records for yourself or whoever might be interested now or down the road. Then there is this other consideration: when feelings are too intense, words seem too small to make meaning; and threading words from the heart across a page is brutal remembrance.

Today I decided I must write. It was exactly six months ago when my mortality or lack thereof came under serious question. Last July 23 I was diagnosed with a huge ocular melanoma in my left eye, my retina was detaching, and I was going blind. The ironies are too great. I had written a book, which is still regarded as a classic text, called *Imagery in Healing: Shamanism and Modern Medicine,* on the use of inner vision for healing. My work for the last twenty-five years has been with and about cancer and its psychological and spiritual dimensions. Saint Lucy, the patron of vision, was on the cover of my book *Woman as Healer.* And over the past few years, I have been senior editor of a medical journal called *Alternative Therapies.* I know virtually everyone in the complementary and alternative medical community and am no stranger to mainstream medicine. I taught and did research at a medical school for twelve years, and I know full well the politics of medicine, especially of cancer.

My own vision has been to bring humanity into the treatment of people in crisis and to do that in any shape or form that I could. At first it was through research that documented the connection between mind and body; later I developed courses in health psychology, taught a gazillion graduate students of one kind or another, and lectured around the world. From the beginning of the complementary and alternative medicine movement, I served on and chaired committees with the National Institutes of Health and the Office of Technology Assessment, the former research arm of Congress. The primary focus was on "unconventional" treatments for cancer, and I've been around long enough to remember when anything that smacked of being avant-garde was called a "quack cure." By virtue of my early association with Dr. Carl Simonton, an oncologist and a fearless pioneer, I have the distinction of having been mentioned on the American Cancer Society's "Quack List" for most of my professional career. My friends in the field have been envious; they considered it an honor, not an embarrassment. With all due respect to those who were harmed by such a listing, I was spared because you had to read the fine print to see that I was an accomplice.

Like a broken record, I voiced my opinion that research and clinical practice had gone astray with their emphasis on chemotherapy, radiation, and surgery and that the alternative medicine movement was pointing itself in the same narrow direction. We heal, and are healed, I believe, by the bonds we form with one another—love, trust, hope, belief, and all those invisible qualities that have lost favor in health care. I wrote as much as I could, and always with the purpose of bringing something of value, and kinder, into health care. These were lofty goals, but sooner or later one just has to take a stand out on the edge of the proverbial cliff or one is taking up too much space on the planet. Or so I think, anyway.

During the past few years, I have been writing and lecturing about intimate and healing relationships—trying, as most writers do, to excavate the territory of my own wondering by giving myself the luxury of becoming immersed in a topic. Be careful, I learned. The Muses have a way of grabbing you by the nape of your neck and shaking you around like a frisky kitten when you set yourself up as an authority on any given topic. "So, smarty pants, you think you know something about this? Maybe you need just a little more postgraduate education."

I recite this vocational history with some humility, for now I have a problem so rare that there are no records in the world of a single case of primary ocular melanoma being treated by so-called alternative methods. In the United States the treatment of choice is either to remove the eye or to treat it with high-tech radiation, sometimes delivered by nuclear reactors normally dedicated to purposes of defense.

I do know something about how the mind and the immune system work and have written extensively on how to integrate this information into treatment programs. The immunology of the eye, however, does not play by the rules of the rest of the body; it is, as they say, a "privileged environment," and little is known about its immune defense system.

Three times I presented myself for high-tech medical treatment, suitcase in the car, expecting to be admitted to the hospital, and each time what I now call the Big Hand reached down and stopped me. Contrary to popular belief, I am sure, I did not reject modern medicine; it rejected me—and that may be why I am still alive. The finest alternative medicine clinic in Europe also refused to accept me unless I first had "that terrible tumor" treated, which meant essentially the destruction or removal of my eye. I was forced to proceed without the protection of medical authority as we know it, to dance on the high wire with no safety net. The view below is fascinating—when I'm not paralyzed by the terror of tumbling into a faceless, bottomless abyss.

Stories, bits and pieces of information, dream fragments, dyslexic notes, crude sketches, telephone numbers of about fifty people who have participated in my treatment (or nontreatment) are scattered throughout my journal, which, at the time, I called "Visions." It is the same and only journal I have used for the first year of vision loss. It is a pretty tacky-looking book, actually. I bought ten of these books with various cheap-looking and semi-ugly covers from a paper company that was going out of business, and if you could see them, you'd know why. Life gets poured out in strange places. On the inside cover, I wrote, "When my Vision returns, my vision will return."

At some core level of trust in the mythic outcome of my life—or anyone's life, for that matter—I know we're all creatures of our own stories and maybe of a story that was written for us at a place and time we don't remember. I don't know exactly where the new vision will take me in the next chapter of my story, but I'm getting some clues that it will be far away from the life I've been leading.

When you are truly in the midst of a process that is so transformative that every cell in your being will shift, the future hides behind a brick wall. I figure if I did know the ultimate outcome, especially if it were really important to me or to the world, I'd probably screw things up by rushing through some important steps, give myself a spiritual or psychological bypass in the process, and miss the whole point.

We'll see. Amazing how often that phrase is used, and it always catches me by surprise, offending me slightly now. When did this journey begin? The Life Force (yes, I do believe that there is such a thing and that it is as tangible as a foot or any other body part) started ebbing away about seven or eight years ago. I read somewhere recently that Francis Crick, of DNA fame, said that now that so much was understood about genetics, you didn't hear so much rubbish about the Vital Force. Guess he must never have felt it depart, much less have it blown back into his forehead. Maybe it was just my imagination, but vampires of despair seemed to be sucking at my soul, and I did not much want to live. Upon waking up every morning, I'd think, "Oh shit, I'm still here." Saint Teresa of Ávila said she had a "dry spell" of seven long years when she felt separated from the Divine. I'm not comparing myself to saints, but it happens to the best of us—months, years when we feel we are orphans of God.

During these years my career as a scientist, an editor, and a professor outwardly marched along at a brisk pace, even though I was on automatic pilot for longer than I care to admit. Classes, lectures, and keynote addresses churned themselves out. In retrospect, though, I was doing nothing of a creative nature and writing no work of lasting value. Thanks to the persistence of Barbie Dossey and Leslie Kolkmeier, my coauthors, the book *Rituals of Healing* got itself into shape and published in 1994. After that, colleagues Donald Rothberg of Saybrook Graduate School and Bonnie Horrigan, publisher of the *Alternative Therapies* journal, still thought I had a voice that needed to be heard, so they interviewed me and got a few of my words onto the printed page. I could not get my hand or mind moving.

My femininity, not my professional self, was under perpetual siege, and the battles left a huge scorched domain in their wake. I love being a woman; I love men and almost everything about them, including the way they smell. All I ever thought I wanted was six children, a home, and a husband who would cherish me forever—and not necessarily in that order—and I was getting prepared. I took four years—that's eight semesters—of home economics in high school, and it nearly disqualified me as valedictorian because it was not "science," but some teachers and parents argued on my behalf because of my high grades.

Many years ago, Norman Shealy—a physician who has an unzipped mind, made major technological discoveries, and then pressed medicine on to more intuitive practices—said the first time we met, "Jeanne, you and I have known each other through our mutual acquaintances and our writings for many years. From the beginning I wondered why you chose to be incarnated this life as a woman."

We were at a government meeting in Washington, D.C., where we were both supposed to be experts on cancer, if I remember correctly. I gasped at his statement. "Why, Norm, what else would I possibly want to be? Being a woman, right now, here, is absolutely the best thing I can imagine." These were, however, still "burning times," a phrase used to describe the several hundred years of European history when being a healer or an early version of a scientist was sufficient reason to have a woman put to death.

Speaking of burning, on the Burn Unit at Parkland Hospital in Dallas, we would see patients come in from all over the country with burns of all sizes and from causes of all types. Mostly they had resulted from acts of violence or neglect. If the burns were not too large or deep, we knew they would heal themselves. All one had to do was help the patients stay clean and comfortable, and nature took over. Skin would just gradually creep inward from the edges of the injury and cover the wound. If the wound was too big, the patients needed help. More skin had to be harvested from their own bodies and used to cover the damage. Sometimes the grafts took, and sometimes they didn't. If they didn't, the patients had little defense against anything that transgressed the boundaries of their hide. On very little people, or for very bad burns, there just wasn't enough self to harvest. When the grafts worked, they left a tough scar.

I've been trying to autograft myself for at least seven years. Most of me is tougher than a boot. But necessary parts of my psyche that are deeply connected with being a wife and a mother are too tender, too raw, to bear any more insult.

At the beginning of this passage into the Dark Night, which got really intense over the past two years, nothing could bring me pleasure—not a sunset, a beautiful home, the warm tile floors on winter mornings (a definite Santa Fe delight), a creative idea, hundreds of wonderful friends, travel all over the world, standing ovations, nada. You'd think a standing ovation would give you a little charge. I was mostly embarrassed. As I said, not a spark of creativity stirred in my bones. I hated my jobs because all I did was sit the whole day long and criticize other people's work. As both a professor and a journal editor, that is what you do, folks. The stacks of paper built up around me—on the floor, in baskets, on tables—and I'd sit down every morning looking at them with the "dreads," otherwise known as that old sinking feeling.

Frank Lawlis, my husband, whom I loved more than life itself, was disappearing before my very eyes, vaporizing more with each passing moment. I had loved him the instant I laid eyes on him twenty-four years ago, and we immediately became professional partners. We even shared a faculty position at a medical school, where the initial consensus was that he was the coach and I the quarterback. He was an academic jack-of-all-trades, and his curriculum vitae was already fifteen pages long, single-spaced, and I had only been out of graduate school for two years, so it was a natural assumption.

Despite my two years as head cheerleader in high school, it was never exactly clear to me what each football player was supposed to do. Other things weighed more heavily on my mind: doing flips without breaking my neck, hopping around and waving pom-poms, and deciding what we girls should yell next. But it did seem that the quarterback was usually the guy who was smaller, pretty smart, fast, and followed the coach's orders. It was the last role that I could not master. I do not follow directions well. Ask my mother.

Frank was trained in West Texas as a researcher and clinician, as well as a football coach. His mentor in graduate school was Beatriz (B.Z.) Cobb, justifiably a legend, and a redheaded, beautiful, delicate, beloved warrior of a woman, who took her "boys" (and they were mostly boys and a few girls) and hammered into their heads the belief that they were brilliant and unconditionally loved (by her, anyway) and could be and do anything they desired. B.Z. was as good a role model as I could find as a teacher, but she was no quarterback or partner. I believe most of her students were in love with her. I know Frank was. He did not say he wanted to marry her. Frank did not question that a woman just might be an authority on something, contrary to the thinking of quite a few men I could name, and I credit B.Z.

For a couple of years after we met, I could not tell where Frank ended and I began. We had the same pale amber skin, were always the same temperature, and he felt as familiar to me as a genetic twin. We were connected at so many levels that when he had a heart attack five years ago, I felt it in my body, which was some 150 miles away at the time. We had what I thought was "an uncommon bond," a connection that intentionally honed our souls. I studied the idea in our lives and with other couples and wrote a book that never got published as well as an endless flow of poetry about our complicated relationship. Someone—and forgive me, I do not remember who—once said that rhetoric was a dialogue with another; poetry was a dialogue with oneself. I needed plenty of conversation about this relationship and did most of it with myself.

Frank and I coauthored a few things and worked together, but not for the same employer very often, and not for long, and we nearly throttled each other while writing our second and last book, *Bridges of the Bodymind*, because we had, as they say, different modes of expression. Actually, it turned out to be a pretty good book, stayed in print for fifteen or more years, and developed a small cult following among academically minded health psychologists. I tout it as an insomnia cure, but it was one of the first of its kind, and the longest enduring book in print on health psychology.

I did not want Frank as a business partner or coauthor, anyway; I wanted him as a lover and playmate, and when we were not distracted, we loved and played all over the world.

Having secrets was part of Frank's nature, and from the beginning of our relationship, it was like reading a book in which the nuances of the plot couldn't be understood because so many pages were missing. Last year I had a dream in which he made a story quilt, and each square was supposed to depict a chapter in our lives. I turned the quilt over and saw that, except for the first square, which had only a single sentence on it, all the cloth was blank.

By around eight years ago, mysteries had started swirling around us like eddies in a tidepool. The secrets gradually got more unfathomable and turbulent, and I felt if I could only get into the center of the cyclone, pay attention, stay focused on simple daily tasks, I could hold us both aground and we would be safe. My perceptions were not deceiving me; I knew what I saw and heard and felt, but not why. By the time we moved to Santa Fe from Big Sur about four years ago, I had expended my quantum of energy trying to keep what Frank called the "Sonny and Cher Show" afloat. I stayed as silent as I could, out of the local public eye, and emotionally and psychologically distanced from Frank. My analysis was that he needed more acceptance for his own talents, to be on center stage without the shadow of my fairly intense presence, and I was tired anyway. That should fix everything.

By last year I realized that I had become very sick but had no clue about the cause. Had a thief come in the night and stolen my life? My passion? The tenacity to live no matter what? Within a week during that year, two of my very intuitive friends had dreams that someone had put a hex on me. Neither told me about those dreams until much later because, they said, the idea was just too strange and I had enough on my mind as it was. I tend to reserve my judgment regarding the Dark Side of the Great Beyond (much preferring to think that all is goodness and light and flowing white gossamer gowns because that makes me happier), even though my friend Larry Dossey had just published a very scholarly book on the subject of "negative prayer," *Be Careful What You Pray For.*

After checking my son into a psychiatric unit for the third time soon after his thirtieth birthday, I was ready to do almost anything to change my life. (My son has changed his own name, and to preserve his privacy, I will change it yet again in this book. I am going to call him Chase, the name I had chosen for a second son if I had ever had one.)

In April of last year Dr. Jim Gordon, a comrade for nearly three decades and director of the Center for Mind/Body Medicine in Washington, D.C. (recently appointed the first chairman of the President's Commission for Complementary and Alternative Medicine, and I am so proud of him), asked whether I was ready to go work in the refugee camps near the border of Kosovo (also known as Kosova). "Absolutely," I said, "if you can help me get a visa." He did. The idea of going to the Balkans did not exactly surprise me.

Four years earlier I had had a strange visit from a woman who insisted on driving down the California coast and up the winding, dirty roads to my home in Big Sur to deliver a message. She was a highly regarded psychic who claimed to communicate with angels, particularly Gabriel and Raphael. They told her that Jim and I were to work together on a peace mission and that medicine would be the vehicle. I respectfully filed it away in my head somewhere, but no, I wasn't interested, and I didn't do "peace," thank you very much. At that time Jim and I had not spoken in more than ten years. Yes, it was a very unusual incident, and no, I don't recall a psychic ever before seeking me out for any reason.

Epiphany: Kosovo

{May 11, 1999}

EIGHT OF US (all but me from Jim's organization and with a variety of professional backgrounds) left for Macedonia to work with the Kosovar refugees, who were in camps along the border or assigned to homes and apartments that could scarcely hold four people, much less the huge families that were their charge. The presence of the accoutrements of war was breathtaking even as we landed in Skopje.

I grew up on army bases and had lived around tanks and guns, but this was different: the huge and frightening presence of NATO vehicles and troops, the sounds of shelling on the border, and always, always the relentless transport of human beings. The refugees were assigned to tents in camps or to buses that would take them to other countries—with seemingly little regard for keeping families intact.

I called Frank every night on a squawky telephone, and I remember some nights when all I could do was sob or stay silent or scream. He was pleased, he said, to hear me come alive again and be passionate about something, even if it was the horror of war.

I was absolutely convinced my life would never again be the same after the Balkan adventure, but just what direction it would take was not revealed to me on tablets of stone. It must be nice when such messages are presented in some linear fashion, or you get zapped in the head with lightning and voices from the spirit world speak. I have not been so privileged.

The stories of my experiences with the Kosovars have not been told, except to a handful of students and as part of an interview that may never be published. And now, as all of us who went have found out, no one is really interested. The experience ripped my heart open—and my eyes—and I knew that for me to survive, I would have to envision the world and live my life in a far different fashion than I had these past years of hanging on a meat hook and slowly twisting in the breeze, like the mythological Inanna, in her journey to the Underworld. Inanna was the queen of the world, boss of the boys, able to choose her charming consorts, but she was eventually stripped naked and her soul laid bare, only to be released from her imprisonment by a compassionate sister.

My life for this past year has also been about children, mourning for my own, watching them self-destruct and me likewise in their wake. To see thousands of ethnic Albanian mothers who had lost their children, some before their eyes in ways so brutal that I cannot bring myself to think about it, brought me midstream into the collective horror. Nothing and everything prepared me for the events in the refugee camps. It was the bleeding of the world soul. It was a crisis about rendering asunder what is most valued—human relationships, families, and cultures.

The most important experience for my own inner life was the last day we spent in the camps. It was one of the heaviest transit days for the refugees—about five thousand came across the border, and many were bused into Stankovitz, where we were working. Others had trekked in a forced march across difficult terrain. I will never, ever forget their faces. I must have made eye contact with thousands of people. Even the children looked directly into your eyes.

There were a few strong young men in the camp (how they got there I don't know, since most were fighting or killed) who were serving as human power for the operation. A huge corridor between the tents was roped off, and as people came off the buses, they were met by the young men with wheelbarrows, their worldly goods (as well as the old and infirm refugees) were placed inside, and they were wheeled down the roped-off area to tents that had (mysteriously, it seemed to me) been assigned to them. As each bus unloaded, thousands of refugees already in the camp surged into the area, looking for family and friends and people from their towns and villages. They were quiet and gentle. There were few reunions. One small redheaded boy who looked as if he had been crying for weeks, and who resembled my own son at that age, ran into the arms of a woman, and that is about all.

Somewhere "back when" I made a contract that I would experience this life as fully as possible, in all its richness, terror, ecstasy, bliss, and awfulness. Faced with renegotiating the contract with the Source, or whatever or whoever is in charge of these things, I always back off. There is a saying from the Sufi tradition, "If you want to face the Great One, you have to learn to dance in both directions." You get steak and ice cream and maggots and rot on your platter, and you have to eat the whole friggin' mess.

I thought, "I need to get into the middle of all of this so that I can understand." Violating the "stay back" commands, I climbed over the ropes and found myself in the middle, facing the incoming flow of hundreds, maybe a thousand or more, ethnic Albanian refugees. In that moment the true meaning of nonlocality, collective consciousness, and the invisible bonds we all share, the terrible and beautiful nature of being human, was densely and thickly real. I think now that I must have said to myself (or maybe I shouted it, which is what I suspect), "No, no, no. We can't do this again to one another. Oh, God, let this not be happening again." I stepped out of the corridor, and within a few minutes Jim saw me as he passed by with a newly deported family. Almost absentmindedly, he said, "Jeanne, you must be getting cold in that T-shirt. Let me find you a sweater." Need I say more about compassion?

It was an epiphany, the larger vision I craved, and one that spun me into another vortex of reality. The experience with the refugees was a validation that life is not about politics or land or possessions or ticky-tacky things, but about how we care for one another. This is one of those platitudes that I'd been mouthing on the speaking circuit with my "Healing Relationship" talks. I always knew the truth of it. Finally I also felt the truth and understood a little more about the mystery and purpose of suffering: it allows our hearts to become connected.

Now I will try to reconstruct some events of a more personal nature. In Macedonia I had been bleeding for about a week, a jumbo menstrual period, the likes of which the world has probably never known. What a coincidence that I was nearly bleeding out at the same time I felt the hemorrhage of the world soul. I had not had a period in four years. The hormones I'd begun taking the previous November, primarily because I could no longer tolerate what I thought were dry eyes due to estrogen deficiency, had caught up with me. I was also taking many supplements that are hormonal precursors, such as DHEA (dehydroepiandrosterone), and had probably about overdosed myself. My DHEA levels were six times the normal level and no one seemed concerned. I will never again take hormones or their near relatives for any reason whatsoever. (This is a personal decision, ladies, and I don't want to get into all that. Maybe it wasn't the pills at all; I could just have been falling apart.)

Nothing much was working properly. I was losing more blood than most people think they have, soaking through one box of tampons and one of pads each day, and it added to the horrors that surrounded me. The latrines were ghastly, a fact not lost on any of the refugees, because cleanliness is an integral part of their culture, and I had to visit them often. These were difficult and tender moments. I had collected an entourage of young girls who followed me, brushed off mats where I would sit, carried my backpack, escorted me to the toilets when I needed to go, and guarded the door. They were beautiful, joyful, full of life, and surely one of the national treasures of the country and one of the reasons the culture will survive.

I was doubled over in pain and taking aspirin, which was making matters much worse by inhibiting whatever clotting my body was trying to do. Joel Evans, an ob-gyn who was also on the trip, gave counsel, settled me down, and assured me I would be OK. We made each other laugh, often, and at what we can scarcely remember. Mostly you had to be there, like when the bus we were on caught fire in the middle of the highway and the doors wouldn't open. (It was just before this event, I believe, after a day of adventure, when one of us had said, "Well, nothing can go wrong now.") The doors did finally open, we dashed out, while Joel directed cars away from us with his trusty penlight, and we retrieved our luggage from the traffic side of the bus.

During the second week of the trip, I had a dream. A mass had come out of me, and I took it to some lab. They told me it was my (what sounds like) orid sponge. (I know now it was "choroid," the area of my eye where the Thing was eventually found.) I asked whether these masses ever live. "Sometimes—but they are not really life-forms. When they live, you can see them: they are the naughty children who run ahead of (or away from) their parents." Certainly this was a prognostic dream that described the metastasis from ocular melanoma perfectly. The tumors metastasize about 40 percent of the time. It is a real fast track out, because there is no treatment, and the life expectancy is three to five months: the aberrant cells do run amok, ahead of their parents.

---◇---

Anyway, back to business. We were doing the essence of alternative medicine, in tents, in the dirt, by NATO tanks, with sounds of shelling in the mountains. We did imagery with young women who had witnessed atrocities that much of the world tries to deny in order to dissociate itself from the awful facts of what humans are capable of doing to one another. We also danced, we listened to the refugees' stories, the physicians did acupuncture, and we massaged babies. For three days we taught seventy-five health-care workers (virtually all refugees and most of them physicians) what we knew about mind-body medicine. Jim and his team have gone back again and again to teach this group, who have since returned home to Kosovo. I went back a year later and was stunned, again, by the resiliency and openhearted goodness of these people. They had taken the rather simple tools of meditation, imagery, and relaxation, modified them, and used them in hospitals, schools, and businesses—everywhere. What I came to believe, though, is that as important as the mind-body techniques are, they are really only the delicate vessel for demonstrating compassion and presence, and for making human interconnections.

On the trip home from working with the refugees, I was exceedingly restless, Joel later remarked. My inner cauldron was being stirred. I prayed for a larger vision for myself, health, my work, my family, everything. On my "What to Do Next" list, written somewhere between Zurich and Washington, D.C., I included several things: (1) We must never assume that the civilized world has divested itself of evil, so that another human extermination would be impossible. Evil is still with us. (2) I must be of service, stay conscious about elevating human values, and use all my gifts to do that. (3) I need more direct people-to-people daily work. This has been a very toxic period for me; it is time now to live the rest of my life. Interestingly I also said (4) I have to hold my vision—which incidentally was the vision of the original crew at *Alternative Therapies,* where, as mentioned, I was senior editor and chief pusher of the paper—and that is a better life for humanity. And (5) I need to stay strong, grounded, and fearless, because I am a role model. I should add that I do not especially like being a role model, nor do I set myself up as one. You just get that way after thirty years in the public arena. The projections are horrific and make me want to hide.

I returned home, my heart wide open, having lost my voice (literally) from a respiratory crisis. In the airplane from Macedonia to Zurich, there were 122 passengers; all but the eight of us were smoking. (Smoking is one solution to serious crisis, and I acknowledged it as such without judgment.) I sat with my inhaler in hand, a scarf over my face; my companions were also gagging, coughing, tearing, and snuffling. I was still wearing the same blue denim jumper in which I had left—our luggage never made it to us until the last day of our stay—and I had grown rather fond of my one dress. Actually I would deliberately have worn it each day even if there had been a choice; the young girls in the camps also had only one dress, and they seemed to love mine with its many pockets and straps. Wearing one outfit for about two weeks was quite a departure for Jeanne the fashion queen.

Papers for the journal in need of last-minute review and words of introduction remained on my lap the entire trip. I couldn't work on them. My hand wouldn't move; my mind was frozen. The field of alternative medicine had been my daily companion for more than five years of editing, and now I had to find a new role for myself. I could not bring myself to try to foster goodwill among researchers and authors, read small pilot studies, get excited about surveys of medical students' attitudes, critique research over and over again. Not that I was too good to do it—I was just no longer capable of doing it.

Homecoming

{June 4}

AFTER ABOUT FORTY HOURS of travel, I arrived in Denver for a layover and called Bonnie Horrigan, publisher of *Alternative Therapies* and my dear friend. Hardly a day had gone by over the past five years when we did not talk on the phone: free-ranging chats about the journal business, metaphysics, gossip, our dreams, families, and girl things—sometimes all in the same sentence. This time we had a little spat. Shit, no, we had the fight of the century. The queens went for the jugular. We didn't see eye-to-eye (pardon the irony) on a thing or two. Or three. Within the week I resigned, and Bonnie generously offered me a paid sabbatical for six months. I was worn out, and she knew it. Once too often I had said to myself, "I can't stand to read another paper." Little did I know that within a couple of weeks, I wouldn't be *able* to read another paper.

Frank could not pick me up at airport because he was seeing patients at New Mexico Cancer Care Center, so I took a taxi for the fifty-mile ride from Albuquerque to our home in Santa Fe and blubbered over the Bonnie thing, although everything was getting mushed up in the vale of tears. When Frank got home from work, he was paler than usual and said he was sick and exhausted. He was always sick when I returned from a trip. I had been sick when I left. Family pattern. He said he had left the telephone ringer on at night just in case I called, and this was a period when he described my son, Chase, as being "on the run" from his carefully orchestrated reality. During these times Chase would call

Frank, sometimes every ten minutes, all night long. Frank would talk him through his panic and once or twice talked him into a safe harbor in the hospital. He also engaged Chase in complex dialogues about the FBI and the CIA, so Chase felt that Frank was the only one in the world who understood his universe. Chase did not call after I returned home, and I neither saw nor heard from him for three months, until I went to his room in a hippie house after my Grim Reaper diagnosis (more—much more—on this later) and knocked on his door. He had no telephone and had dropped out of the medical system and away from his friends by then.

On this return, sick or not, Frank was obviously happy to see me alive, engaged, and passionate. He had ordered me a beautiful Cadillac—not a new one but the dealership's best, a fast, well-engineered little jewel. This is what Texas men do for their women, for reasons that are not entirely clear to me, but it seems to be in the genes. I'd been ragging on Frank for several years for selling off my Seville, with its leather seats and wooden dash and fabulous sound system, for little more than you'd get for scrap metal and buying a piece of new tinny junk that I refused to claim. As they say, "Big Sur eats your car," and it had done a number on the underside of mine, so truth be told, the old Caddie needed a lot of work. Maybe I could have put it on blocks in the front yard, used it as a planter or something. Anyway, it was part of our good-natured sparring, but Frank vowed he would redeem himself on this one. As it turned out, the car would probably save my life—I have an idea some cars do that—once I became forced to drive the highways struggling with rapidly altered depth perception. You really need only one eye to drive, but it takes a while to get the hang of it.

Vision Quest

{June 19}

A STRANGE, METAPHORIC EVENT took place in mid-June after I returned from the Balkans. Frank and I were planning a camping trip in August with our friends and close companions Barbie and Larry Dossey. Now I want to say at this point that this book may read as if I'm doing a lot of name dropping. That's because I am. During the most intense period of my Descent into Darkness or wherever the hell I went, beginning most seriously in about a month, almost everyone I can think of in the business of healing reached out to me.

The Dosseys were like a lifeline. They are pure gold. Unlike some other famous and semifamous whom I need not name, the Dosseys tell the truth, keep their integrity, and their work will endure forever.

I do not go camping, although I used to sleep outside in Big Sur all the time. Outside is good, unless it is too hard or cold, and New Mexico is usually either or both of those things. This, however, was the second disastrous night out on the land. (I will relate the first occasion in one of my "flashbacks" a bit later in the book.) Frank and I had decided we'd better test our new sleeping bags and mats, and we went out around sunset to the large rock formation on common land behind our home. The view is spectacular, and the land is holy, if hard. As if we were going on a traditional Vision Quest, which is a common cross-cultural form of initiation or wisdom seeking in wilderness settings, we took stone fetishes (mother bear and coyote) and water. I also took a candle—just in case. It was unusual—a candle within a candle made of beeswax—and I figured it wouldn't blow out in the wind. A new friend, Jim Lake, a psychiatrist in Monterey whose life would synchronistically intertwine with mine, had given it to me after attending an imagery workshop.

I realized after the sun went down that I was not feeling well at all and guzzled a quart of Perrier without once removing the bottle from my lips. I awoke around midnight, greeted by the strangest weather conditions ever witnessed in June in New Mexico. They were so unseasonal that even now I think it might have been a dream. It had started to drizzle, and the fog was dense. Fog on a high mountain in the summer. The wind was blowing in gusts and swirled the rain and fog around but did not improve visibility. I told Frank I was going back to the house, but I don't think he heard me. He seemed OK: he had his face peeking out of his sleeping bag and looked comfortable and dry. I took the bear fetish, matches, what was left of the candle, and a scarf with fringe and metallic threads. I am possessed by the goddess of outfits and figure you need to have a little touch of something unusual, just in case. Thoreau was simply wrong when he said no occasion is worth buying new clothes. Maybe this is sort of like when you were a kid and Mom or somebody told you to wear clean underwear "just in case" you got in a car accident and they took you to the hospital. Why the scarf, I don't know. It didn't go with my navy Polo sweats at all. Eventually I wrapped it around my head to keep my ears from freezing, so I did make a fashion statement as I slid and stumbled through the wilderness—as if anyone cared.

There was no moon—nothing. I headed in what I thought was the direction of the house. It is very easy to get disoriented on the mountain, even in the daytime. I saw a pile of deadwood that looked familiar, so I went toward it—but the incline felt too steep. I grabbed onto trees, lit the candle, and walked a while longer. Finally I saw a recognizable rock-lined path and turned left—obviously the wrong direction. I saw something that looked like a white dead animal and walked around it. It must have been a reflection off some quartz; the mountain is made of rose quartz and very little else. I turned off to the left and walked uphill again. Another bad decision. I had to crawl in the steep places to keep from falling and grasped onto trees. The candle eventually died, and I threw it down. Many times since I have walked that land trying to find it in order to resolve some of the mystery of my whereabouts that night, but to no avail.

I had no clue, vision, or landmarks. I quickly learned to crawl under thick clumps of trees because they seemed to lead to smoother places. There was not a single house or road in sight. I must have walked an hour and finally heard highway sounds but still could not identify the landscape. Finally the houses and shopping center of the township of El Dorado came into view, and I decided to go in the other direction, which is where I believed I lived. The white Orthodox Greek church was there in my face. It is on exactly the opposite side of the mountain as mine: if you could tunnel through the mountain from our house, you would connect directly to its back door. I thought about spending the rest of the night inside curled up on a pew, but it was really very, very cold, and I heard peculiar clicks and bleeps and wasn't at all sure someone else hadn't taken refuge during this eerie dark night. I walked out to the highway instead, made sure I was on our road, and then walked the two miles home. Animals, big ones, went crashing through the bushes. I wondered whether they were two- or four-legged.

It was probably three or three-thirty a.m. by the time I saw my adobe palace at the top of the mountain and what looked like orange balls flying above it. Oh, God, maybe Frank woke up, found me missing, and got scared and sent up flares or something. The balls moved very fast—jerking around. Later I told Frank I thought they must be the lights of dirt bikes. He said, "Not likely. It was after midnight, and there are no roads up there." We don't know what they were. I later learned from stories of the Southwest (*Witchcraft in the Southwest: Spanish and Indian Supernaturalism on the Rio Grande,* by Marc Simmons) that witches in New Mexico were believed to take their night flights in these not uncommonly sighted fireballs, which swooped and whirled and sped out of sight. Often in these tales the enchantress loses the sight of one eye during her night voyaging and is obliged to borrow the eye of her pet or familiar. After the incident she appears with the round, strange eye of a cat or an owl. (This would make for quite a story, but I'm not inclined to dramatize my life along these lines to make it more interesting. I'll give it some thought after I've had time to catch up on my paperwork and ironing.)

The night sky had cleared by the time I reached the house, and all the constellations were brilliant. I have never before or since witnessed such a spectacle. There were more stars than darkness. When I got home, I decided to get out of my dirty clothes and put on a pretty gown in case Frank came in. I never knew how much he noticed these things, but he might have. Again, it never hurts to have a touch of style.

I slept in the guest room (it has better ventilation in the summer) and had the nosebleed of my life. Nothing clotted, and I tried to stanch it with towel after towel until I finally dropped off to sleep. When I awoke, blood was thinly caked all over my face. Pillows and sheets and the velvet duvet were bloody. Well, after having lost nearly all my blood in Macedonia, I must have been registering empty by then. All of it came from my left nostril, less than a half inch from where the tumor in my eye would be diagnosed the following month.

Then there was this recurring dream that did not feel like a dream but like something out of a time warp. In this dream the blood is really a circle of something gone awry—like a broken necklace (that's the only way I can explain it)—and I have to tell people it was not a nosebleed but something else. Something disconnected. What a dream. I got exhausted having to repeat myself so many times: "It is not a nosebleed. It is something disconnected." Standing my own ground on the diagnosis I was going to get in just a few weeks would be a challenge that would require every bit of stubbornness in my constitution; it would also involve exhausting repetition that was ignored, just as in the dream.

On the other hand, maybe I just accidentally ate rat bait, I thought with my usual grim humor, medium-to-good knowledge of physiology, and insight gained from my position as chairperson of our house's rat and mouse infestation committee. This is what rats do after they eat rat poison: they drink like crazy, run around a lot, and then bleed out.

I did not have a single scratch, which would be truly impossible even in the daylight in the cactus- and brush-filled terrain. I never fell, and my soft-soled shoes, like Indian moccasins, felt the way. Frank returned around five A.M., when it rained again, saying he had come the safe way on the road to the water tanks and still had fallen down twice. He was badly scratched. I can't figure this whole thing out, but it was a metaphor, a message of things to come—that much was clear.

I wrote, "Will try to retrace—find out about the candle, the lights, etc. Has something to do with my strength, madness, children, and the weird property we have. I thought several times, 'This is a hell of a way to make friends with land.' But I did learn: my feet learned the terrain; the trees helped me. I was totally without vision or direction, and it was OK.''

This is a story of triumph through darkness, and it does have a positive ending. The dream was about having to argue over and over to explain that a physical symptom was not really what it appeared to be. Something was disconnected. I did walk in darkness, but I discovered how to find my way home over dangerous and unfamiliar terrain and arrived with no injuries whatsoever. There was also a biological connection between this bleed, several others, and what was eventually diagnosed as a tumor in my eye. There has to be a relationship. It all happened at one time, in one body, and now I will never know the details, but only the larger story, the metaphor of where the Vision Quest has led. The incident on the mountain was the dress rehearsal for a play that was about to begin.

Business as Usual, More or Less

{June 21}

WE WENT OUT to Father's Day brunch at the very best place in Santa Fe for such things, and I could not gag down a bite. Then I flew to San Francisco to teach for Saybrook Graduate School, where I've been a faculty member for longer than I can remember. Saybrook runs one of the oldest "at a distance" Ph.D. programs and has been accredited for a long time. We have been good to each other: the adult students nourish teacher instincts, and the pace fits my own—episodic splotches of human intensity, interspersed with periods of hermitage. I usually chair dissertations rather than teach courses and have negotiated myself out of faculty meetings so that I seldom have to be there in person.

After the walk, crawl, scuffle, and bleed episode, I felt like a piece of crap. I was dizzy, unstable, and had started another little period, and whether I was losing vision or not, I don't know. One hardly ever squints to check on monocular vision. Something was definitely going on, though, because in San Francisco I canceled my rental car and took taxis instead, something I had never done before, and it cost me a non-reimbursed bundle of cash. Five days later I left California, went to Texas to give a talk and a workshop for the Texas Nurses Association, visited with family, and then flew back to California to attend Saybrook's graduation, after which I returned to Santa Fe. This is craziness, and the reason why I am a 1K flyer on United Airlines. That means 100,000 or more miles are invested in my little body each year, and the year of my near demise was no exception. Flying through several time zones a week is not unusual for me. The cells in my body must regard chaotic biorhythms as the norm, and my threshold for discomfort must be high. In retrospect, I was very sick, sicker than a dog, but at the time it was hard to distinguish severe fatigue and jet lag from "very sick."

Why didn't I go to a doctor? I'm scared of them, for one thing. A study in the *Journal of the American Medical Association* showed medicine (mistakes, blunders, and reactions to drugs) to be the third leading cause of death in the U.S. of A., right after heart disease and cancer. And by then, I had so darn many things wrong with me that I figured I was about toast anyway. If I was on my way out, I wanted to keep most of my parts, and given my current symptoms, it seemed likely that my uterus would be the first piece of me selected for removal.

Initiation

{July 4}

AFTER I RETURNED from my travels on June 26–27, I was high and
excited, as I usually am after teaching and lecturing, right before I crash
into a mixture of boredom and doldrums and work-overwhelm plus
overwork in the home environment. On the weekend of the Fourth, I
had a dream, a command—something that I desperately needed to get
all the sorrowing Black Madonnas out of the house. People had sent
icons, pictures, and postcards of this brown or black archetypal woman
to me from all over the world. I'm not sure why. I felt absolutely
haunted by them, by what they signified, for my own life and for the
women of Kosovo. It didn't help that we are living on the edge of a
burial ground, which was discovered after the house was built and while
the land in front of it was being leveled. Many small tribes lived in that
area at one time, and the remains of their fire circles are up past the
rock formation of the famous Vision Quest–nosebleed night. The best
guess is that the burials probably resulted from one of the many raging
epidemics and included quite a few children.

In the middle of the night, I grabbed all the Black Madonnas I could
find and ran down the stairs. A ceramic pot on the stairway seemed to
jump toward me and crashed. It did not fall backward the way it would
have if I'd bumped into it, and I can't figure the physics of this out.
Frank, who had been sleeping outside on the porch with our dog,
Yoshie (as he did most of the summer until Yoshie died), came running
in and cleaned up the mess. The pot hit my head and left a wound over

27

my left eye—just in time for publicity pictures to be taken that next Monday for an interview I was doing for *Alternative Therapies.*

At this point I remember having seizure-type flashes in the left hemisphere of my brain and sensations behind my left eye. I walked back up the stairs thinking, "I'm going to have a fuckin' seizure, right here, right now. Then I'm going to faint and die." It was probably my retina detaching, but then who knows?

◇

A week later, on Sunday, I found Yoshie dead behind the bench where we were having morning coffee. He had apparently simply died, just then, and was still warm when I touched him. There was a small trickle of blood on his mouth. His timing had always been perfect, and that is characteristic of the breed. This beautiful 110-pound dog came to us from Samoyed Rescue in San Francisco when Frank needed a four-legged, unconditionally loving friend and left before our lives got too distracted to give him much attention. I was so afraid he would die during one of our long times away, and he was already quite old for a big male Samoyed.

His spirit lingered, and for months I could almost see him out of the corner of my eye, in the shadows, snoozing in favorite places where he'd dug into the cool earth. For the week after his death, a white cat came to stay in the yard and disappeared as quickly as it had come. Yoshie was cremated by a gentleman who considered it a spiritual privilege to do this for people who loved their doggies, and he brought me roses when he returned the ashes.

At the suggestion of my artist and writer friend Lee Lawson, I decided to take the week off from food. Lee is one of the girlfriends who was always there. She paints what I write about, and I write about whatever she is painting—just by coincidence, of course—and she is an intuitive and a dreamer par excellence. Several precious pieces of her art adorn my walls, so I am always surrounded by the essence of Lee. Her book *Visitations from the Afterlife* is as inspired as her art.

I decided to do a six-day lemon juice fast. This is really a pretty nasty business. All you do is drink lemon water and maple syrup and a dash of cayenne pepper, and eventually the kitchen gets so sticky from blending the concoction that your shoes make great sucking sounds when you walk across the floor. Fasting, Lee reminded me, spurs creativity. She knew well that I had lost my visions over the past years.

That Friday I got the headache of the century (and a little period again). I was really sick and shaking. I also had a brown thing, bruise-like, on my arm. Ugly, spreading. Having a little too much medical knowledge for my own good, I begin to suspect a platelet or clotting disorder of some kind. Or had the air miles, the constant return to eight thousand feet, where we lived, the anti-inflammatories, the supplements and herbs, the acidic fasting, the lifestyle, just crept up on me? Frank gave me a chiropractic-type adjustment on my neck and a quick massage on Saturday, and said, "Wish I knew where you got those bruises." I did, too. They weren't bruises; they didn't hurt.

————◇————

The headache from hell continued unabated, and by Sunday morning I could hardly move. I was supposed to drive to Albuquerque to catch a plane in the late morning to Riverside, California, to give a talk for the American Cancer Society and then return that night. The bleeding was continuing, too, and the bruises were spreading. The only thing I knew to do was to get into the wet sauna to take away some of the aches. Frank opened the glass door and stared at me for a long time. His mouth trembled and twitched. This is one of his expressions that conveys some intense emotion, but I know not what even after all these years. I sat on the bench, holding my head in my hands, shaking.

About an hour before I was supposed to leave, Frank left for the airport to fly to Dallas and spend some time visiting with his son. He called later in the afternoon to see whether I had gone to California. I was still home.

I had gotten dressed and put my slides together for the presentation, but as I pulled onto the highway, my car stalled, and I had to call the auditorium in Riverside, page the organizers, and cancel my talk.

————◇————

It would accomplish nothing for me to air a laundry list of what Frank and I did and did not do during this healing crisis. I believe he simply did what he could and offered what he had to give. I received what I could and stifled my pleas for help because it embarrassed me to feel so incapacitated. Sickness is not a familiar territory (except in others with whom I have worked), and I did not recognize severe illness in myself even when it had become a monster lurking everywhere. A small voice kept whispering, "Hey, if you guys can't learn to take care of each other, who can? Get with the program here." I would have argued strongly against Frank's staying home, this time or anytime, and he did not offer. I was always afraid that if I did ask, he would refuse or else stay and be surly or far too quiet, and then I'd just feel guilty. Frank was remarkably noncritical to me about what I did or said or how I looked. The trade-off—which served me well, usually—was kind of a benign neglect. During unstable times he retreated and I advanced— with my mouth.

We were about to face one of the two major health crises of our life together. The first was his near-fatal heart attack and the aftermath, when everything changed—our home, jobs, friends, and on and on— and not all in a positive direction, if you want my honest opinion. For the past years in Santa Fe, we had made some modest headway in beginning new lives at midlife. Still, when crisis really strikes, we act like two cats in a bag.

—————◇—————

The headache that had begun on Friday did not go away until Tuesday. By that time I knew that something was wrong with my left eye. I spent most of the week worrying; experimenting with different lights, glasses, and contact lenses; and trying to decide how much of my visual field was missing. When I finished a nine-hour stint revising an interview for the journal, the world of sight was only light and shadow and wiggles. My vision in both eyes has been poor enough. Since the age of eight I've been considered legally blind without glasses or contact lenses. The possibility of total loss of vision in one eye was alarming and threatened my work and mobility.

Medical Mystery and Maybe the Black Widow: A Retrospective Investigation

AT THIS POINT I'd like to push the pause button and put the narrative on hold so we can travel back in time to the previous summer. You see, it's occurred to me that maybe the Eye Thing started long before the symptoms I've been describing and maybe it is not exactly an Eye Thing at all. So bear with me here for a couple of retrospective chapters, because a few points need to be made about the complexity of the body-mind connection and how symptoms don't just appear out of nowhere, and it would behoove us to look at the larger story.

That summer, about a year before the onset of my full-blown symptoms, I nearly offed myself twice, once in a dental chair and once out in the backyard with what looked like some kind of bites—probably from a black widow spider.

I had elective surgery for bone grafts in my gums, and it did not go well. I have definite problems with drugs of all kinds, and anesthesias are always dicey. As soon as the anesthesia entered my veins, I could taste it and feel it whack me on the left side of my head. My right side went numb. I got extremely cold and stayed that way. I asked the dentist to try to clear the anesthesia, but it didn't clear and never really knocked me out either. He finally turned off the blood pressure monitor, even though my heart was pounding. Best to just ignore it. I don't remember pain but instead great concern that I would leave in a body bag. I had to breathe oxygen for at least twenty minutes afterward and felt half-conscious for the next four hours.

I trace to this event one of the steep descents of my downhill slide toward the nether regions. This doc may have overdosed me (although he said he only gave me a small amount). Then he blamed it on epinephrine. He and my dentist had a consultation. Epinephrine was probably part of the problem, but the poison hit my head long before the local injections with epinephrine, which is really adrenaline, the stress hormone. (A little note here: Epinephrine is strictly for the convenience of the medical personnel. You don't bleed so much, and it makes their work easier. It is hard on the patient, though, and I have since refused it.)

I slept a lot the week after the gum fiasco. Frank said, "The surgery pickled your brain." God forbid, I thought it was menopause, and here it was just the anesthesia.

That same week something possessed us to sleep outside in the backyard. You'll recall that in an earlier chapter I told you about the *second* time we slept out—the night of the Vision Quest–nosebleed the next summer. Well, this was the *first* time we had slept out, and the circumstances turned out to have been about as unusual as they would be the following year. I woke up with at least three huge black-and-brown bruiselike things—probably black widow spider bites, the natives said—and I should have been taken to the emergency room immediately. The spiders may have joined us—or me, at least—because we had put our sleeping mats on old lawn chair covers that had been draped over the woodpile, the black widows' favorite habitat. Now, who would know that? One big mark was on my foot and another on my arm. Actually there may have been several on my left arm. The one on my foot took six months to quit hurting. The one on my arm looked awful: you don't get a bruise like that without being hit with a baseball bat. You certainly wouldn't sleep through it.

I was very, very ill for two days. I felt poisoned with a neurotoxin, as one might after a black widow attack. Bang, ping, poing—neurons clanging. The closest I'd come to this was a very bad psychedelic mushroom adventure. Certain mushrooms are poisonous and slightly neurotoxic, and that is why they give visionary experiences, but I just felt my hardwiring shorting out then, as well as after the black widow bites or whatever they were. That morning, as I was waking up in that half-asleep, half-not state, I heard my father trying to get into my door, and whatever it was, it was no dream. I heard the clink as he messed with the lock. I screamed and screamed. He'd tried to get into my door once too often when I was a kid. I didn't know where he was then, but I was not going to let him come to get me. This dream still frightens me. If "dead" is wherever he is, I won't go there. Or maybe he was coming to make amends.

The editors from the *Alternative Therapies* journal were supposed to meet at my home the next morning. I was very sick, probably dying, and not exactly sure from what.

I had slept outside the preceding night and would do so again the following summer. Both times I had dreams that were not dreams and was close to checking out for good.

———◇———

Late that July, a few days after the spider's work, Melinda "Mo" Maxfield and I went to Rancho la Puerta in Mexico, a magical health spa guaranteed to fix whatever ails you. For years I have crawled in on all fours, panting and exhausted from my goofy schedule, and leaped out at the end of the week, a new (or at least resuscitated) woman. You start off before daylight by climbing a mountain, and I mean fast, and then the regimen intensifies if you so desire.

Mo is one of the finest women on the face of the earth, and no one much argues the point. She was my student many years ago and is now one of my very best friends. Her research on the effect on the brain of the type of drumming associated with shamanic healing practices has become known throughout the world. She has an expansive knowledge of healing in its many domains and a superb generosity of spirit. Her historic estate is an oasis, and I always figure if I can just get there, no matter how difficult the crisis, all will be well. Mo is one of the "girl-friends" to whom I have dedicated this book, and she was the master anchor of my healing process. Her earthy feminine wisdom grew out of Texas tolerate-no-bullshit roots, and she is the truth-teller among us. She doesn't have MOHAVE on her license plate for nothing, and I love her dearly.

I had to wear long sleeves the entire week at the ranch because I looked like a victim of wife abuse. Mo said, "You don't get marks like that on your body unless you've been clubbed." Now that I'm thinking about it, during this time—even the first day or two at the ranch—I had what felt like seizure activity in the left half of my brain and over my left eye. It was so intense that I was afraid to listen to Mo's shamanic drumming tape for fear it might provoke a full-blown seizure. Normally I use the tape on a regular basis, as that kind of drumming has always been used to "journey" for information and healing. I was also aware that it was 110° in the shade, and I was having chills, so I got into the hot baths and sauna. Sweating like a pig may have saved my life, as it caused me to exude whatever ailed me.

Sometimes when you hurt, you just don't know where it's coming from. My foot hurt. My face hurt. Mo hurt, too—she'd just had foot surgery—and the two of us dragged ourselves around like the Hunchback of Notre Dame. We didn't make any new friends this time. We mostly hid out, bitched, and ate Advils.

This hurting intensified over the following month. Then I went back to Dr. Gum Graft, and he found a "cyst" (actually an abscess around a failed root-canal job). It couldn't drain and was just growing. Antibiotics. It got better; I didn't. I was morbidly depressed, and now I can recognize what must have been a low-grade fever that just never went away. I dissociated from physical symptoms in order to survive my lifestyle, so I didn't think too deeply about any of this, except how to get from one place to another, including the grocery store.

Dark Flight

BEFORE RETURNING to the summer my symptoms erupted, I'll extend this "flashback" for one more chapter—to consider a series of losses during the previous autumn, winter, and spring that also form part of the larger story and may well have contributed to what was to become the Eye Thing.

In September, about nine months before I had the first physical signs that something was wrong with me, and the day before Frank and I were scheduled to leave on a trip to Paris, my birds disappeared from their cage on the front porch. I am still trying to make sense of this terrible event, because it was the harbinger for the darkest time imaginable, and for tragedies beyond my comprehension. I got both birds as babies and hand-fed them probably longer than necessary because they and I enjoyed the ritual of scooping up mushy baby food, which they swallowed and splattered all over with chirps of delight. They kept me company in our isolated setting in California and paced the cycles of my day with their natural rhythms. Often I would bring them into the room while I was writing, and they would sit for hours on my shoulders.

Pet birds are like children, as any bird lover knows. Persephone, or "Perci," the African gray, was as smart as a three-year-old, had an interactive vocabulary, and could speak in both Frank's and my voices—but mostly mine, since I did most of the talking around her. She would call "Frank" in my voice, and say "What?" in his, which gives you some idea of the typical nature of our interactions. Or she would go "*briiinng*" like a telephone, say "Hello," and then chortle, "Heh, heh, heh."

She was in many ways like my thirty-seven-year-old daughter, Lee Ann—talkative, persistent, inquisitive, and merciless in her tenacity when she set her mind to a task.

J.C. (short for "Jesus Christ," named by Frank in defiance of all the goddess figures in the house), an umbrella cockatoo, was my white angel (and no one else's, I might add, since he did and could bite to the bone). His squawk could be heard for a couple of miles on a quiet morning or farther when he did his cockatoo thing of calling the flock at sunset. His favorite expression was "I love you," which was enough for me. He, like my son, was occasionally a mama's boy—endearing and cuddly, but only when he felt so inclined.

Taking them was a senseless act. J.C. was truly of no value except to me: a raccoon had torn off one of his wings when he was a baby. The mysterious disappearance happened when I took my mother and her husband, Will, out to brunch. As we walked down the sidewalk near the plaza in town, a white and gray feather fell from the sky and landed in front of me. "Ah," I thought as I picked it up, "my birds are sending me some kind of message."

As we drove up the driveway before noon, Frank was barreling down the hill in his green Nissan. When we passed, he stopped, backed up, rolled down his window and shouted, "The birds are gone."

"What? Did you go look for them?"

"No, I thought you'd taken them someplace."

"Where would I possibly have taken them?"

I was shocked by the news. You don't exactly take birds out or borrow them, any more than you would a fish. Birds shit all over everything, especially if they are scared, bite people, fly away if they can, and these guys could chew up a chair in minutes.

This was not a random theft. It was done by someone who knew our habits or had been watching the house for several days. My mom's car was parked in the driveway while we were gone to brunch. You don't rob a house with a strange car in the driveway in broad daylight unless you know whose car it is and how many people were in the house, who left, when they left, and when they were likely to return. Or at least I wouldn't think so. We lived on a cul-de-sac in the middle of nowhere. Doors were unlocked, and money was visible through the windows—I was sorting my foreign bills for the trip—but nothing else was disturbed or missing. Whoever did it knew how to handle the birds, or there would have been feathers around from the capture. And why did it happen the day before we left instead of while we were gone?

I suppose the birds could have gotten out, but the cage was locked from the outside because J.C. could escape from a jail. I bawled for a while and called their names outside for the rest of the afternoon.

About six weeks later, when I returned home, I called a reporter at the local newspaper to do a story in case someone had seen the birdkids. It was on the front page. I had one call from a nurse who did home health care. She said the mother of one of her clients was bragging about her new African gray, "Paco," and she knew they had no money for such a thing (they cost about three thousand dollars). She told me where the woman lived in the *barrio* and where she sold crafts on the street. My daughter, who is a "dreamer," also dreamed of the birds often, and once she saw their location, in a Hispanic section of town, off a major street named after a saint, and behind what looked to her like a double-wide mobile home or a home that was not quite a home. The setting was almost identical to the location the nurse had described.

In one or another of these revelations, the word *bruja* was mentioned. A bruja is a witch in the Spanish tradition. Bad juju. I decided it would be unwise to try to locate them myself and remain convinced that at least one bird is still alive. I've left their large cage filled with their favorite toys open on the front porch for the past two years just in case they are returned.

These events marked the beginning of major losses and were a smoky mirror of what was to come. I do not fully understand how the birds fit into the metaphor; I only know that they play a major role. In trying to make sense of the senseless, I have wondered whether their names were not chosen through mere happenstance or cleverness, but to be a reminder of eternity. Both Persephone and Jesus Christ were figures who supposedly died to life as we know it; went underground, so to speak; and then saw the heavenly light of day. Persephone's agonies and adventures during her time of darkness are legend. What went on with Jesus when he was in the crypt could be a great chapter that remains unwritten. I doubt he just lay there, still, cold, and waiting for the time to pass.

Wherever the birds are, they are still my allies and remain in my dreams. I believe when we humans provide sustained care for any creature, we are loved in return and linked by some invisible, compassionate web forever.

Over the years I have established a reputation as having decent intuition, and I have had precognitive dreams since I was a child, as my daughter does now. Like many highly receptive people, I put up barriers so I would not feel too much or be confused about what was coming from me and my life and what was being projected at me from others. This was particularly true for my children. I have always felt a keen linkage, like electrical circuits, connecting them to me, even before they were born. Why would it be different afterward? So-called ESP information is so nonspecific that it is best not to be too quick to act on it. Sometimes I absolutely *knew* one or the other child was seriously in harm's way, and would go berserk and pace the floor, only to find out afterward that the kid had merely been anxious about something and not in a car accident or whatever peril I had conjured up. I mention all this because, during the coming year, I did *not* pick up on any dire circumstances surrounding either of them.

Frank and I went to France as scheduled and met Mo and Judy Ostrow. (Judy is another of the girlfriends on the journey to whom I owe my life and sanity, or what is left of it. She has taken many trips with me: we travel the world doing almost anything to have fun and have thus far managed to stay out of serious trouble.) I hated France; I hated the thoughts in my head. We could see the Eiffel Tower out our window, and I still hated Paris. The walking tour through the Basque country was a pisser. Every step hurt. The rooms were too small, the people on the tour too arrogant, the food too redundant. I forget all the travels, but I went home and then, after five days of downtime, back to Germany.

———◇———

I found out during the brief interim at home that Lee Ann had gone blind on the fourth of November. She would become quadriplegic by the end of the month. No one could say for certain, but it may have been a reaction to the influenza vaccine she'd received the same week or a first presentation of multiple sclerosis or God knows what. Her lifestyle was like an old hippie's, and between that and the ton of chemicals she was on, I wasn't sure she would survive. She was scared. We all were. When I saw her that December in the hospital, she couldn't have weighed more than eighty-five pounds, and her little arms and legs were as cold as ice. I took a plant decorated like a Christmas tree to her hospital room, not realizing she could see neither it nor me.

By New Year's Eve she had reached a nadir. I was awake all night thinking I heard the phone ringing, waiting for a call from the emergency room or the police—which would in fact become the story for the next few months. As I look back, I realize that Lee Ann actually showed surprising strength. She got on task, obtained welfare assistance, and got medical care. To this day I am in awe of her survival skills. I dared not take her out of California because of the economics of her care. California, for all its faults, has a magnificent welfare system compared to most.

Then Chase, my beautiful son whose looks once outshone Matt Dillon's, had an apparently psychotic episode in mid-January. He was picked up screaming in the middle of the night, in the middle of the street, wearing a tinfoil suit. Cocaine was suspected, but the problem continued long after the coke was supposedly gone. He was never adequately diagnosed or treated.

I made so many trips to hospitals to visit my children that I've completely lost track of the details. More than a year afterward, I was surprised to find an unused airplane ticket dating from that period. I must have changed plans and forgotten, but then again, my plans changed often, and God bless Kay and Mary Ellen at KD Travel, who can also be counted among the girlfriends who have managed to ship me around on a moment's notice. Also I felt so supported by the legion of women who were no strangers to drugged, sick, and/or dying children. Unfortunately there are many of us, and nothing in the book of life prepared us for these events.

I usually stayed with Mo during these emergencies and drove to visit the kids from her home. There I had the privilege of sleeping in the beautiful white lace canopied bed of her daughter, who had died from leukemia more than ten years before. Seeing no end to it all, I bought a laptop computer so I could continue to work no matter where I landed. It lived at Mo's for one full year. Many things were left there—

books, art supplies, gowns and robes—as it became a halfway house between the dramas of life and death.

Getting on and off airplanes to see my children during that terrible time is about all I can remember. I called Frank from a layover in Phoenix and told him I couldn't go on, I just couldn't face another hospital visit. That was it. I was returning home. "You'll make it," he reassured me, and of course, I did.

I spent a week working on Chase's rehabilitation with Mel, my first husband and the father of my children. Our efforts were to no avail at that point—except that Mel and I had a wonderful reconnection. My apologies to him were long overdue. I had always loved him and wanted him as my friend, but we no longer served each other well as mates after sixteen years of marriage. The pain I created by leaving him was unthinkable and unforgivable. He has lived a life of integrity, and I am so very proud of him and his actions of true humanitarianism. Because he married Frank's ex-wife, we are in each other's lives forever anyway, but I can't go into that story just now. As they say in scientific literature, "It is beyond the scope of this paper."

Mel and I parented these sick adult children as best we could. We did the laundry, fixed up their living circumstances, and got them groceries. I played Martha Stewart for Lee Ann, enjoying both it and her. We made a zillion trips to Kmart (not my favorite place, dahling) for things to put things in. We bought a new floor fan because the one she had lacked a protective cover—the blades spun around while a blind girl stumbled across the room. This woman had been living in the back of her truck for more than a year, and sometimes, when she was lucky, in a moldy trailer in a campground. But you know what? I'm with her. I'd rather be outside in Big Sur than almost anyplace in the world—but with a few more amenities, naturally. She is a sweetie even if she lives a strange life on the dole.

The situation with my handsome son was less cordial, to say the least. Some of the doctors on the psychiatric unit knew me, and Chase was afraid I would use whatever influence I had to get them to keep him there. He was absolutely correct, and I would have if I could. He was in no condition to be released after the requisite seventy-two-hour hold, and although there are quirks in the state laws that may protect patient rights, those laws also make it more difficult to protect truly ill persons from themselves. Chase will not forgive me for many things, among them the fact that when he was sixteen, I had him arrested and immediately put him in a treatment center after he'd robbed us, disappeared, dropped out of school, and become addicted to speed. The police in our drug-infested Texas town understood the situation well and were kind, but they gave him to me to take—wherever—and we made the trip to the treatment center alone, together. I believed then and still maintain that speed opens up a part of the soul to evil forces, and if there is such a thing as demonic possession, I saw it in Chase's face. This was someone, something else—not my son.

That spring was spent with Chase alternately in the hospital, running from the FBI and the CIA, and trying to go to a computer tech school. He did come to Santa Fe once, overdosed on Haldol, which was not his fault, drooling, shaking, dragging his feet, and smelling awful. I quickly called Marius and Alexandra Wirga, our psychiatrist friends from Poland who are doing residencies at the New Mexico State Hospital, and they immediately prescribed antidotes. Again, I wonder how other people cope without such resources. Even with the best of the best available, this kind of crisis sears one to the quick.

Chase has always been secret and sensitive. He saw "auras" around people when he was three years old. I didn't even know what auras were. I don't see them, for sure. "Mama," he would say, "you need to fix me some breakfast right now."

"Why right now?" I asked.

"Because," he said, "my rings are turning yellow."

I asked what rings, and he pointed to a space about an inch from his hand. Turned out he saw rings around everyone, and they seemed to change color depending on moods. Once, when Chase was about five, I happened to mention his unusual abilities to a friend at the Institute of Noetic Sciences in Petaluma, California, and he sent someone who was knowledgeable about such talents to Fort Worth to visit with Chase. I don't know what good this did, but Chase never forgot it. The investigator concluded that Chase carried a strange energy around him, and he tried to show me the invisible substance of Chase's energy in his hands and then threw it to the ground and stomped whatever it was with his feet. I was trying to be an open-minded but skeptical scientist, interested in the anomalous phenomenon, especially as it pertained to my children, but had to roll my eyes anyway.

Chase told me when he was about nineteen that he quit trying to see the auras because it just irritated him. He knew things about people that were disturbing, and he saw little use in having the information about the rings. Chase has had a secret fantasy life, and has always been one for drama, so I cannot separate outer experience from his inner and very private material. Only Frank interacted with the worlds that the rest of us could not perceive. He listened to what we all considered delusional systems and gave Chase advice on how to protect himself from the threats and taunts of the voices that he heard, he said, "24/7." Chase remained convinced that Frank had insider information, and he was the only one Chase trusted with his realities. I was in no condition to protest because it kept me obliquely in touch with my son.

———◇———

This period was the worst time of my life, and I had absolutely no defenses for it. Platitudes about building character during difficult times were offensive, since I had about as much character as I or anyone else could stand for the time being and was operating strictly in survival mode. It was hard to face each day, braced constantly for the possibility of another telephone call. I hurt all over, had strange fevers. I slept in about four-hour stretches, often sitting on the living room couch, never fully awake or asleep.

The house itself seemed haunted. Pictures flew off the walls, objects fell off of tables and onto the floor, and there were places around the kitchen where the dog absolutely would not walk. Frank said that nothing like that ever happened when I wasn't there and chalked it up to the usual unexplained phenomena that he says have followed me around for as long as he's known me. Well, maybe.

One afternoon soon after Frank had left for a trip to Dallas, I was consulting the I Ching. (The I Ching is a method of "inner looking" from ancient China that has always been helpful and accurate for me, despite its arcane language and imagery. We each pick our own inner-looking devices, and this one just happens to be mine.) I heard what sounded like an explosion upstairs and discovered that the chandelier had fallen onto a glass table. I am still finding splinters throughout the house. It seems difficult to imagine this happening due to natural causes because bolts would have to have been manually unscrewed. I do not remember what *I Ching* turned up, but it got my attention at the time.

Since we are at quite a height on a huge bed of crystal, and lightning frequently makes our house shimmer, the electromagnetic energy must be uncommonly strong. Paradoxically, the area feels healing, and we are undoubtedly privileged to be the first inhabitants on sacred ground, between a burial site and a ceremonial site.

If the kids were going to die, though, I felt obliged to die also and be with them. Wanting to accompany them to the afterlife to make up for not being totally available in this one might be a mother type of thing. Who would want to live if you lost all your children? Going to the Kosovar refugee camps, though, was an inspiration. Whether they want to or not, mothers do go on living after their children are dead, and my children were still alive, albeit very sick.

I was scarcely functioning and certainly not creative but was still tending to business, doing public lectures, and so forth. People told me how good I looked even when I felt the worst. Either they were being kind, or I must give credit to the "little work" done on my eyes (girl talk and what most of us decide to do after people comment once too often on how tired we look). Since the past November, when my daughter was diagnosed with the Unthinkable, Unknowable, I had been losing my long, multicolored blond hair, which had been my trademark, and feeling stringy-haired and ancient. My hairdresser even noted that it looked as if a big chunk had been cut out on the back of my head, like when you take a hair sample. He called the other hairdresser over to look at it. "Yep," he agreed. Gross.

―――◇―――

With 20/20 hindsight (if you'll pardon the expression), it would seem that this recent period—during which my system had barely survived the twin insults of a hellish anesthesia reaction and a near-fatal black widow spider attack, followed almost immediately by a series of critical losses—could well have paved the way for what would become the Eye Thing. Let's return now to where we left off two chapters ago—to the point at which the intensifying symptoms were about to be given a name.

Grim Reaper Diagnosis

{July 23}

THIS MORNING I finally became convinced that I had a detached retina after reading *Introduction to the Principles of Disease,* a tome that will scare the bejesus out of you on any given day. During my walk to check on the garden, I couldn't find my footing; textures and colors were an unpredictable kaleidoscope. When you are losing part of your vision, it is hard to figure out what is wrong. I asked Frank to drop me off at the hospital emergency room on his way to work: it was the only way I could see an ophthalmologist immediately. He agreed and came back after an hour or so. The emergency room was not yet open for emergencies, it seemed, and I was still sitting outside the door when Frank got there.

We were supposed to leave with Barbie and Larry Dossey the next week on a camping trip, and I had a four-day workshop in Colorado before then, so I knew if I needed something fixed, I'd better get it done quickly. We were going to get dropped off in the wilderness and ride horses for a week. The first and last time I had ridden a horse was twenty-six years ago in Mexico, and I kept yelling, "Oh shit."

Mel, my then-husband, finally hollered back at me, "Try 'Whoa.'" Little family joke, but I was getting very nervous about bouncing around on the back of a horse for eight hours and having my eye come loose.

I'm scared to death of doctors and modern medicine, as I mentioned, and seeking medical care on an emergency basis meant I'd crossed over from the fear zone into panic. "After all those years teaching at a medical school, how can you be afraid of doctors?" so many ask. "My point, exactly," say I.

This day initiated the journey into hell and was what I know that most people who are diagnosed with serious disease experience in some form or another. The doctor in the emergency room was a very nice, cheerful guy, who showed up forty-five minutes or an hour after the official opening for the day. By that time I was wondering whether I should start writhing in pain or something to get this process going. My presenting problem was written down as "eye strain."

He dilates my pupils with nasty chemicals, peers into my eyes, and then sends me to the ophthalmologist across the street. This young man, who looks about eighteen years old (as so many do, and you wonder how they had time to get through medical school), puts more chemicals into my eyes to dilate them, and I figure I have the largest pupils in town. Maybe this is not so bad; Italian women used to dilate their pupils with belladonna to look sexy and mysterious, two qualities that are distinctly better than ugly and scared—which I feel I am. He (doc number two) confirms the detached retina and says I need to get to the Big City doctors as soon as possible. Like today. As you may have guessed, I need to keep much of this description anonymous because, as per usual, I don't want to hurt anybody's feelings, and I damn sure don't want to go to jail.

I know that all these guys must have seen the bloody mess in my eye but didn't say anything because they were passing the buck. Paying their bills strained my goodwill and integrity because I felt deceived.

I finally got sent that day to the Big City, suitcase in hand, expecting to be admitted to the hospital for a procedure. Before leaving, I called the Dosseys because I needed their support and vast medical lore. They gave their love, and it carried me like a magic carpet through the day and the next year. As I've said, they are a lifeline, the voices of sanity and compassion.

This is the first of several times I expected treatment at the hands of modern medicine and was sent home instead. The clinic is a dump. All the patients are scheduled for the same hour. I, the Princess Goddess, am not liking this at all and am not really understanding the system or how I fit into it.

"But I have an emergency and need surgery, and my appointment is for three o'clock."

"Everybody's appointment is for three o'clock. Have a seat."

I am the youngest there and about the only one not needing a walker, a wheelchair, or a portable oxygen tank. I do get special treatment and am bumped up in the queue. Chemicals go in the eyes one more time. The Eye Man looks into my eye; gets real quiet; relays some cryptic information to his assistant, who scribbles some marks on a circle representing my eye; and then asks if I have anyone in the waiting room with me. Although all my oars are not in the water by now, I am not stupid and realize that this is not a good sign.

"Yes, my husband is in the waiting room, but let's just get on with it."

This strange memory crosses my mind of a young African girl who was telling her story about her clitoridectomy in a newspaper article. She knew what was coming and said, "Hurry up. Just get it over with." I feel the same way.

In the kindest way possible, he tells me my eye is full of blood, there is a very large tumor, an ocular melanoma, and I have a sixty-forty chance of survival. If it has spread, the average life expectancy is three to five months. Given the tumor's size, the probability of its having spread is high. I ask what color it is, and he says, "yellowish with spots of blood. But melanomas don't have to be brown, you know." I tell him about the eyelift, as well as the bleeds and the infected tooth thing, both about an inch away from that eye, and he just shrugs.

"No, there is no way any of that could be connected. No one ever comes off the street with an eye looking like that." That's what he said—twice. I didn't get it, but assumed he was validating a diagnosis that was never again to be contested by anyone who saw me.

I finally fetch Frank, and he comes into the dark cubicle of an examining room and does his vacating number. I've seen that look before, like when he is bored in a lecture, scared, or embarrassed. I saw that look twenty years ago for the first time while he was waiting to go on a local television talk show in Dallas, right after Chef Jim had demonstrated how to fry some kind of meat. I knew he was anxious then. Frank yawns and then yawns again.

"What's wrong?" I ask.

"Nothing, I'm just sleepy." Shrouded. Gone fishing. I can't tell whether he is really about to fall asleep, so worried that he dassn't show it, or just interested in something else. To this day he says that he knew I'd be just fine and that it was a misdiagnosis, so maybe he really is just sleepy. I hope he is right, and it is of some comfort that he maintains this position in the face of my terror and paralysis.

This is not what was supposed to happen, though. As he said later, "In one day everything changed." Yes, it did. He had previously insisted that I would live to be very old and he would not. I was never so sure about this, but up until then he had been the sick one for sure. Heart condition, thyroid disease, gout, hypertension, unstable blood sugar, vertigo—you name it, he had it. It was a standing joke among our friends how much time Nurse Jeanne spent monitoring his vital signs—something he didn't need and I could just as well have done without. It simply goes to show you not to be so sure about your old-age financial planning and who will be left behind.

At the Big City Eye Clinic, Frank sat behind me quietly in a cluttered back-room laboratory while I had two sonograms done—the second one because the tumor(s) appeared to have no mass inside. It made no sense then or now. They looked empty, and Eye Man thought the machines were busted. The technician argued with him and said that the machines were just fine and had recently been calibrated. "Do another one anyway." I got a few more layers rubbed off my corneas. Same results. He said I needed to be seen by another eye doc with better machines on Monday. But then he must have changed his mind, because he referred me instead to the MRI (magnetic resonance imaging) center and a specialist, Dr. Shithead. (All kidding aside, his real name has escaped me forever.)

The Eye Man really tried his best—felt terrible, no doubt, about giving me a death sentence—as he arranged for a bunch of appointments the next week. I pressed and pressed for more information. I asked whether a needle biopsy might confirm the diagnosis. He considered it for a few moments and then decided against it. It was a lousy idea anyway, and I don't know why he even let it cross his mind. If the Thing was cancer, a biopsy would dangerously spread the tumor cells. For a brief moment in time, I just wanted it gone, the Bad Thing out of my body. I now understand why people are so willing—even anxious—to have their parts removed when they get the diagnosis of cancer. I wanted to get information, treatment, and on with it all as fast as I could.

I did ask Eye Man for a prescription for sleepers. I figure if you can sleep and take the edge off the pain, you can deal with about anything, and these are the two major benefits of modern medicine. He asked with a quizzical look, "Why aren't you sleeping?" I said, "Because I seem to be going blind, and it's got me a little worried."

The women in the office, one by one, come up and hug me before we leave. "I am so sorry," they say with tears in their eyes. Two mention including me in their prayer circles. I hear one say, "Oh, God, no. How awful." I am very touched but not encouraged that this bodes particularly well for a prognosis.

It was the beginning of the end of me, for sure. Fourteen pounds dropped off my tiny frame within two months, and I bemoaned the years I'd wasted worrying about being too fat even when I weighed less than 120 pounds. I called friends and family because I wanted their prayers. I said I would not allow anyone to tell my mother I was sick until three days after I died because she would be so anxious I'd have to pluck her off the ceiling. But I relented, partly because I needed her tenacious support and partly because I needed her to take me to appointments the following week. I could still drive but knew that the batch of docs would put chemicals in both eyes between seven and twenty times in a single day, and that does make one a menace on the road.

———◇———

Here I am again, talking about events instead of more important things like feelings. I think I was in shock, and shock serves a very useful purpose: it enables you to keep on keeping on. My first inclination, though, was to dread an untidy dying process. "I just don't want to leave in a mess" was among my first sentences announcing the Thing in the Eye. Within a few days I'd decided that maybe my next chore was to model a graceful and conscious way of dying. That didn't seem too bad.

A "final exit" was a possibility, but none of the available methods seemed too certain, much less final. Sometimes even with the best intentions and a jug of pills, you wake up brain-dead. Given my screwy metabolism for drugs, I might just get wired on 150 Dilaudids and want to dance, the way Rasputin did when his enemies fed him enough poison to wipe out the Russian army. With my doctor buddies and a visit or two to Mexico, I could come up with a potion—which I would use unstintingly if I started peeing in my pants or getting real ugly. I later learned that this is called Plan B by those who have encountered this particular decision-making crossroad. Now I know better than to think like this, but such thoughts do prey upon one's mind.

Into the back of my mind also creep thoughts of Ginny Hine, my mentor and friend, who paved the way by taking her own life, with great ceremony and awareness, when she felt she had done the work she came here to do. "Ginny, where are you now?" I wonder. She promised to stay in touch after she left, but aside from a power outage the moment she died and a cold breeze when I thought of her later, I have not felt her spirit waft my way, and I am wondering what happens in the hereafter if you take yourself out.

I revisited one of my favorite authors, Keri Hulme, who in a quasi-fiction piece, *The Bone People,* writes of her diagnosis of stomach cancer. She is a woman after my own heart, and I often think of her story. As I returned to it, I was struck by the similarities. She asks medicine only for pain relief and rejects hospitalization. "Primarily," she tells her reasoning, "I forgo control over myself and my destiny. Secondly, medicine is in a queer state of ignorance. It knows a lot, enough to be aware that it is ignorant, but practitioners are loath to admit that ignorance to patients. And there is no holistic treatment. Doctor does not confer with religious who does not confer with dietician who does not confer with psychologist. . . . [A]nd the attempted cure is often worse than the disease." Instead, she opts for isolation and silence, finds a place to die in and stocks it with groceries. She brings in two crates of whiskey and a bottle of extract of hallucinogenic mushrooms—a painkiller of unknown strength and potent effect. I could do this—it would be my style. But what would I substitute for whiskey and mushrooms? She makes notes:

> Little febrile clots of words
> that choir in earfuls
> humping off the page.

Yes, I could do this—make notes, see God, and visit the ancestral spirits. Hulme's protagonist, the part-Maori Kerewin, and probably herself, crawls out a month later, cleans her filthy self off, devours a meal, and notices that the huge growth and knife-sharp pain are gone. Well, that would be something, too.

What was bad during this time were the hysterics whenever I mentioned death, especially to family. Most people were putting me in the grave already; I could hear it in their voices. My sister-in-law asked the futile question, "Why do good people who give so much to the world have to die and the bad ones live?" It was a compliment. My brothers wanted me to come to Texas and party hearty—a sure sign of deep affection, and I appreciated the offer but was not at all sure I could keep up with them.

I did not come out of the gate fighting, nor did I exactly fall down. There were some decisions to make: I wasn't sure how much I wanted to live or whether or how, and I knew that such information was not going to pop into my brain overnight. Things had been going downhill for a long time, and the Grim Reaper diagnosis did not exactly perk me up.

Demon Diagnoses

{July 25}

SUNDAY. I WAS SCHEDULED for a photo shoot, for crap's sake. Athi Mara Magadi, a portrait photographer of some renown, was doing a gallery showing on "Santa Fe Originals," forty women who had "broken the mold." She is wonderful; her photos capture character, which most of us had instead of beauty. "Well," I think, "I can either cancel this sucker and act like a sick person or go ahead and act as if I'm alive." She made me feel beautiful anyway; the photos came out great. I'm smiling. My eyes look normal.

Mom and Will showed up while I was getting the pictures taken. Crisis is Mom's forté. She is a bulldog when it comes to nagging any system into compliance, and she had her work cut out for her this time. But I couldn't make her happy. She spent considerable time telling me why I should "put up a fight" and live. I had so much to give, blah blah blah. I was sick of giving, didn't she get that? Why would I want to do more of the same?

I have intensely disliked the idea of "fighting" disease since I began working with cancer patients. Most of the time it is introduced half-heartedly to please the next of kin. It is also a symptom of a prevalent mind-set that medicine is practiced in a war zone and we are all little soldiers trying to live forever. A fearless-fighter attitude is necessary even to survive the system of medicine, but this was not the time to bring it up to me or force me to say I wanted to stay alive at all costs.

I tried to talk to Mom about what I was thinking, about "chosen

51

karma" and "given karma," although certainly not using those words. But I do think about that. So much of my life has been a surprise, unplanned, charmed, directed by some other force—given karma. How did a girl like me get into the right places and at the precise times to live such a rich life? Defies the odds. What spider wove me together with the men and women in my life? What energy guided me away from a miserable, nomadic, abusive childhood to the place where thousands would be praying for my health, because, they said, I was loved? I couldn't have planned this life; I couldn't even have imagined it. How did I manage to have two children who became my greatest source of sadness and my best teachers? Who was I to say that that other Force was not now directing me toward the Conference in the Sky? You see, I just don't know about these things and distrust people who claim they do.

Mom's solutions were quick and dirty: put the adobe palace up for sale *tomorrow* (since I didn't really love it, and it was so big that everything rattled around in the massive spaces), and forget my grown kids who can't get their lives in order. Furthermore, she gave Frank a talking-to about his care of me and (I suppose) significant words about his lack thereof.

The following day brought more trips to bigger cities and clinics from hell. An MRI and another opinion. The MRI cost seventeen hundred mostly nonreimbursed dollars, no one but a radiologist ever looked at it, and no treatment decisions were ever based on the brief written report. I can read. It said ocular melanoma was the likely suspect, but because of many other factors, such conditions as bleeding of the uvea (the pigmented layer of the iris) or a cyst could not be ruled out. The uvea bleeds like any other place in the body and makes a mess that is often confused with melanoma. Since I'd been bleeding and had had a cyst right under the area where the Thing was found, I figured someone ought to have at least made a note of that information in the report. No one did, however.

We waited in Dr. Shithead's office for three hours for the radiologist's report. You can tell I'm not pleased. Once again a slew of us visually challenged people had been given the same appointment time. Since hairdressers and dentists have figured out how to schedule people so they don't wait all day, I am curious about this peculiarity, which I faintly remember from the clinics at the county hospital in Dallas where I worked.

My eighty-four-year-old mother stood at the receptionist's counter the whole time. "You can have some coffee and take a seat, ma'am," someone said about every fifteen minutes.

"Nope, I'm staying here until the report comes in and the doctor sees my daughter."

It never arrived. She got in the car and drove to the MRI center to pick it up. That's Mom. I'm sure the radiologist wrote it on the spur of the moment and probably while she was banging on his door. I was in another waiting room with my good eye staring into space and my not-so-good one turned inward.

The worst of the bunch so far—actually from then on out they got much better—was Dr. Shithead (and his slimy-handed associate), who recommended a bomb specialist who uses a nuclear reactor to smoke your eye. S.H. also said I should be checked "every inch" for metastasis: "They can do great things now with liver pumps."

I know better. This is medical baloney. Sticking a chemotherapy pump into the liver of a person with metastasized ocular melanoma would be about equivalent to burning someone more slowly at the stake, and God knows I have some faint memory of what that was all about. You might last a little longer, but it wouldn't be worth it. I feel no need to express my opinion further on this matter. Why in hammer hell would I want to be checked over every inch for metastasis when, if metastases were found, the likelihood of my surviving until my vacation trip to Kona, Hawaii, would be slim?

I asked Dr. S.H. if it could be anything else but melanoma, and he screwed up his mouth and shook his head. I was getting used to that expression.

"Are there ever any spontaneous remissions?"

"Never."

Wrong, again, Shithead. Go read a book. Sorry for the sarcasm. I am not a happy camper at this point. For such a rare tumor, there is an exceedingly large number of remissions without any known treatment. But of course, this information reveals itself to me only much later. Maybe Shithead was not so bad. Maybe my reaction to him was just a case of "Kill the messenger of bad tidings," so I forgive him.

Two of the oncologists who work with Frank, Tim Lopez and Rhonda Fleck, a husband and wife, look at my MRIs, offer consoling words, and get on the Net to search for treatments. Tim tells me with some assurance that he sees metastasis only in very sick people, and I am obviously not sick, but I am getting weaker and more scared by the moment. I know (and he does not know I know) that he treated a young mother who died only two weeks before from the same condition. She was quite healthy until a month or two before her death. These two physicians, who had no "real medicine" to offer in my case, sent me an aromatic box of my favorite things—herbal bath salts, shampoo, lotions, and potions. The definition of medicine, or "that which helps or heals," is expanding—and so is my appreciation for physicians who are also healers at heart.

At this point I could not do any healing imagery. I disbelieved the diagnosis, for one thing. My imagery simply could not embrace the idea of a tumor in my eye. My consciousness can travel throughout my body—into my hand, my heart—but it did not, would not, enter into the Thing in my eye. I had no dreams, no intuition to speak of. I knew it was something, but not what. I was calculating all the health problems I had had recently, and it could be that I was just falling apart.

The physiology of the eye, which I had carefully memorized in graduate school, was long forgotten, nor did I look it up until six months after the diagnosis, violating my own best advice to patients: "Learn about the nature of the problem or disease so that you can imagine the healing process."

Again, I remembered the dream of "disconnection" after the Vision Quest and the purported nosebleed and tried to sort out what it all meant. What is disconnected? An eye or a life?

———◇———

Before leaving for California for a few days of alleged vacation, I spoke on the phone with Robbie Gass. He was my "main man" in the beginning and a great source of inspiration and information. Robbie is a psychologist whose music is known all over the world. His recordings of chants from various spiritual traditions are a reminder that voices in harmony make celestial sound. I turn them on full blast and sing in my car, in my bedroom, and in airplanes, and they are a staple in my training sessions, because it doesn't matter whether the language is Sanskrit or Latin or English, you know you are singing to God.

More than ten years ago, Robbie had had the same diagnosis—ocular melanoma—and was also told that it was huge as a barn and life-threatening. He, too, was praying for a teacher and went blind in the desert. Robbie had a six-month-old son at the time, and I think that for that and other reasons, he chose life much more quickly than I did. He talked about the sheer terror of it all, and that made me feel better. I was utterly terrorized, and maybe that was OK. Terror was unfamiliar territory, and it helped to have it named. He also talked about his re-covery—canceling his seminars and trainings for three years, meditating for hours at a time in a dark place, making a new connection with life. He had many resources to draw upon in his healing: friends, spiritual practice, the ability to spend days in retreat, his great love of nature and music. I was envious.

"But, Robbie, what would I do if I quit working? I'd just sit around feeling sorry for myself."

"Jeanne, we need to have a little talk!"

He was right. There must be more to life than working, but in the past few years that had been the only item on my agenda. I did need to think about getting a life. Or else. Not right then, however, not while in shock mode.

Robbie left a song he wrote on my answering machine later in the fall when I was in the depths of awful decision-making time. I curled up on the floor and cried when I heard it and have never erased it to this day. We agreed that we are a club—people with ocular mela-noma who are trying to live consciously. He said he felt absolutely healed before his radiation: he had worked with many healers and each time felt well. I learned this to be true: each healing session, prayer, ceremony, call, card, or gift brought healing to me at a new place, an-other level.

The calls and prayers, dreams and visions, rolled in. Healing net-works and prayer chains were formed. I was astounded at the energy directed my way. My eye is surely the most prayed-for organ in a living being. I don't know how the word got around so fast, but it did. Stan Krippner, a fellow faculty member at Saybrook and my inspiration as a teacher, was a constant source of prayerful support. He is also one of the busiest humans on the face of the planet, but he managed to make a connection with me several times a week by E-mail or calls and notes and cards. Stan took to heart a message he received many years ago from Spotted Fawn, wife of the famous Native American Rolling Thunder, and he tells his story in Lee Lawson's *Visitations from the Afterlife*. Stan was in Mexico, and Spotted Fawn appeared to him in a vision and thanked him for being present with her, saying how important it was to be with people you love, especially if their lives are threatened. Unbeknownst to Stan, Spotted Fawn had died that very night.

Larry LeShan called that first week. Larry is a prolific writer, smarter than God, and a national treasure. He was the first to draw parallels between quantum physics and spirituality (*The Medium, the Mystic, and the Physicist*) but is probably now best known for his book and lectures entitled *Cancer as a Turning Point*. Right out of graduate school, the very first year I worked with cancer patients, I had a dream that I had been assigned to continue his work, and I protested mightily that as a woman, I could not follow in his footsteps. But I did follow up on his work, often to discover that what I thought was an original idea, he had already proposed. We met in person almost ten years later, and I had the audacity to ask him to marry me in a future life.

"My dear, that makes the prospect of death quite pleasant. Only with the next turning of the wheel, we will do it in the fast lane. Harrods, a Bugatti, the Riviera." Sounded good to me.

He reminded me of what I already knew—that the only way you stay alive after a serious diagnosis of cancer or anything else is to find your visions. I told him I had lost mine, at every level. But I simply could not jump into how to change my life right then. Although I didn't want to disappoint him, I could not say what he wanted to hear. I was just trying to make it through each day, plan for the medical stuff, get my head in shape, and pack for a trip to the unknown. It was premature to reorganize my whole life at that point, and I feel guilty because I have avoided several conversations with him, even though he was motivated only by love and care for me.

More than a year and a half later, Larry and I met again in California at a "Turning Point" conference at Stanford. He was his sterling self and reminded the audience of nearly one thousand people that cancer is a turning point only if you decide to turn. Then he had a private little talk with me in which he minced no words or feelings. I apologized for not returning his calls, but it had taken me almost a year to find my way back into life. I thanked him for his caring and told him my eye was surely the most cared-for, prayed-for organ ever.

"It was not your eye that was being prayed for; it was your life. You are a marked person. Not everyone is, you know. You have been marked to do important work in the world. I've been watching you for a couple of years. You were unfocused; we were all afraid you would die."

"Don't you think that we are all marked to do something with our lives, that we have some seed that begs for expression?" I asked. It was a rhetorical question and not answered to my recollection.

"You are not finished yet."

"Oh, Gawd," I think. "Don't you ever get finished? A condo on the golf course? Who are all those people with cameras on the Santa Fe Trails tour bus? They must be about my age, and they look as if they've finished their work and gone on vacation permanently."

Angeles Arrien, one of the wise women of the world, called me and said she had awakened in the middle of the night and gotten a message that I should call Bill Stewart. Bill is the director of the Institute of Health and Healing and was chairman of the Department of Ophthalmology at California Pacific Medical Center. I had forgotten that Bill was a vision man, although I knew he was a visionary. It was his institute that had sponsored my imagery training program in California, and his staff worked long hours to get it fully accredited for physicians, nurses, and psychologists. Bill helped get me into a referral network on the West Coast, which was a relief because my extensive support system was clustered in that area.

Carl Simonton, my oldest friend on earth, the pioneer of the mind and cancer, was always there. His first words were to remind me to pray to all my ancestors. He continues to use healing words to frame and reframe my experiences, without which I would likely be a dead doggie by now. Carl and I have been in love with each other for more than twenty-five years. Through marriages and divorces and all of what life has put on our plates, we are there together in some way.

When we met, we were married to other people than we are now, and although getting caught kissing in the sauna may have accelerated our divorces, it did not cause them. We have never had an intimate relationship, and now that we don't have so many urgent hormones (well, I don't, but he probably won't admit to any deficiency!), we sit blissfully for hours, hold hands, even fall asleep together on the couch, and share what is surely unconditional love. Sometimes he is a Bad Boy and I am a Bad Girl, but there is nothing to forgive because we just *are*. We teach in Europe, *Same Time, Next Year* sort of thing, and catch up on each other's lives.

That night when I called him and said, "Carl, I hoped never to have to make this call," he knew right away. "Last year in Germany you said you were tired of living. I can imagine me saying that, but never you. I knew something was very wrong. You've always carried so much light around you, and it was growing dim." This was right after my daughter's diagnosis, the loss of the birdkids, and in the midst of an oozing, virulent depression. Well, he wasn't doing too well either. Our moods and fortunes cycle remarkably in sync, and both of us had spent the two weeks we were in Germany sleeping as much as we could between our training sessions and cocooning in our respective rooms. Thoughts of going home were about as pleasant as the idea of walking back through the gates of Hades, and I only perked up one day when I spent eight hours on the streets of Garmisch doing "shopping therapy" and had to buy a duffel bag to carry back home a pair of boots and a beautiful, stylish, very European yellow knit skirt and matching sweater. Little did I know that this was to be my near-death outfit—or my return-to-life outfit, depending on your perspective. Almost one year later I had it on for five days when the Thing in my eye erupted like a volcano and I could not get out of bed in a hotel room in Washington, D.C. The coincidence probably doesn't mean squat, except that everything is connected, and these were happy clothes, bright yellow, and the color of the life-giving sun.

During the first call after the Thing was diagnosed, Carl gave me an assignment: Write down ten things that bring you joy and are life-giving. I forgot the assignment. He called every day or two. "Have you written it down yet?"

My response usually was something articulate like, "Do what now?" Classic. Shame on me. With each call he reassured me that he was certain I wouldn't die but that I did have choices and changes to make—which, of course, I knew, but not what they would be. Renovating my life would not do the trick; I had to reinvent it, and dying would be far easier, I soon found out.

Eagles Everywhere

{July 28}

MORE CALLS AND PREPARATIONS to leave for California. Sandy Ingerman, one of the legions of girlfriends, a Santa Fe neighbor, and author of *Soul Retrieval,* did special work for me today. She is able to travel to mysterious worlds and pluck back parts of you that have escaped because of fear or losses or trauma. This old medicine is believed to heal wounds of a soul nature and reinstate your personal power. I knew that it worked and that she was the best. During the soul retrieval Sandy journeyed to the Underworld, the shamanic regions, and found an eagle for me. The eagle became a guardian spirit—giving me keen vision and direction. As I think of Eagle, I am reminded that Bonnie Horrigan and I both dreamed of eagles the night we opened the *Alternative Therapies* journal office in Santa Fe. We bought two—a carved wooden one and a funny stuffed puppet. The latter guy sits staring at me as I write.

People say, not without kindness, "You have so many resources. What do other people do who are not so fortunate?" I am scared shitless and foundering and feeling all alone most of the time, so what *do* they do? Twenty-five years ago it broke my heart to see cancer patients sitting in a line of chairs, waiting for radiation, chemotherapy, or they knew not what. They were all dying, not from cancer but from fear. Nothing has changed. Maybe it's getting worse. Now they're confused as well because, in addition to regular medical treatment, the alternative or complementary therapies receive heavy press, and everyone and no one seems to be an expert. It is time for this bad old business to change.

59

◇

The following day we headed for Big Sur, California, our former home and where I'd left the part of my heart that loves the ocean combined with the drama of earth and sky. Frank drove the whole way, and I remember placing a pillow on my lap, putting my head down, and sleeping for hours at a time. He drove to and from California doing his usual rendition of a bat out of hell. We decided that the only thing good about the trip was that I had lost so much vision in my left eye and was so distraught that I didn't look at the speedometer and nag, which was my usual modus operandi in situations that I felt were seriously life-threatening.

Going to Big Sur first instead of to more doctors was a decision we made with mixed emotions, because there was still so much uncertainty—in our minds, anyway—about the diagnosis. We were restless, or at least I was. It was certainly not a vacation, but I felt the urgent need to do some inner work, and it was as good as it could be under the circumstances. We stayed at Ventana Inn for three days, mostly in a beautiful bed with soft pink sheets and huge pillows next to the fireplace. The familiar ravens and blue jays swooped by the window, and the smells of the ocean and the season of yellow grass in Big Sur were poignant reminders of what I had left behind.

Frank held me for hours and hours every day and tried to do the imagery for me. He imagined birds pecking away, breaking up the Thing.

"Mel is in there also, complaining that I'm not doing this right." That, of course, would be so true of my perfectionist ex-husband. Afterward Frank wrote down the imagery he "received" for me:

> Eagles, eagles everywhere, showing you vistas, swooping down valleys, showing you the life above the turmoil. Eagles urging you to soar with them, letting everything go, wanting you to join them in knowing this other reality. Eagles pecking at the decayed aftermath of growth, taking the life from it, leaving the rest scattered. Eagles peering in your eye, questioning the reservations about joining them, J.C. joining their ranks, showing you his love. Eagles from their lofty height see the connection from the eye, from the heart, the poison that is generated from hardness and fear. They want to

free you from the suppression. Eagles want you to fall in love, many times, to fly with your passions, to free your heart to soar. There are smells to excite the heart, juices to drink. There are no choices, no fears. The loves you will have will have no criticism. Take the changes and trust your path, your wings.

Frank's warm presence was comforting by my side. He is a big teddy-bear man, and cuddling was one of our very favorite activities. I remember the first night we ever slept together, and he was stiff as a carp.

"If you are going to sleep with me, you'll have to learn to cuddle," and I flung my leg across his and gave him a demonstration. He was a quick study, and we became masters of the cuddling arts; we cuddled to celebrate, to mourn, and just to get warm. We could flip over in tandem and never lose contact. It was the first thing he had asked of me right after his heart attack, and I crawled into his hospital bed and settled in among the wires plastered on his chest.

My own healing work could only begin with him, my constant companion for so long. He is intuitive and inventive and even dreams of medical treatments and gadgets that are unknown to science and are eventually discovered by someone else.

In the professional training groups we co-led for many years, we always talked about transpersonal imagery—images that were sent across time and space to another. There is plenty of research to support the idea that we affect one another by our thinking with awesome consistency in ways that can be both healing and damaging, depending on the intentions behind the thoughts. If anyone could do transpersonal imagery and have it affect my DNA, it would be Frank.

Even so, the eagle imagery had a slightly odd flavor to it, like when you bite into a piece of fish and think, "Something is off here." Frank volunteered that the birds weren't the best imagery because they were messy eaters and left a bunch of junk lying around. That's what it felt like: I was losing vision at an accelerating rate, and whatever gook was floating out and causing the retina to detach had increased. There was something else deeply disturbing about his images, and my heart, already in spasm, grew harder: he imagined me going or wanted me to go on alone.

Snowballing Support

{Late July and Early August}

DURING OUR STAY at Ventana, the healing network grew. I asked for and got a telephone session with Jean Houston, a woman whose creativity and generosity are boundless. She worked with Robbie Gass for five days during his "health challenge" (as they say, and this is another phrase I could stand never to hear again) and assisted him in staying in a healing trance. I found her to be sensitive and helpful. She gave me some of the best advice I ever received, and I later shared it with many people who were in crisis.

She said, "You go find at least six people to hold the 'trust' space. You can't do this right now, and this is where you need the most help." Eventually I invited the assistance of hundreds or maybe thousands of people who wanted to help me in some way to be tethers to faith and trust while I was consumed by pain, fear, and the unknown. Jean said I was in "Calypso time," a time outside of time. She said I needed a *big* rest and should take at least three to six months off.

"Is this what people do?" I wondered. "Where would I go? What would there possibly be to do?"

Don Campbell, author of *The Mozart Effect,* called and talked me through a meditation, much as I had done for him when he had a brain aneurysm, which he describes in his book. This was truly transpersonal imagery. We were on the telephone, several hundred miles apart, both of us went into trance, and I went into his brain. What I saw frightened me, and the imagery he was using would quickly have caused serious harm if it had had any biological impact at all. Together we found a sound and an image that he felt were essential to his healing. I am unable, or don't try, to do transpersonal imagery very often, rarely on the telephone, and have never been so directive as to tell people to stop their images because those images will kill them. What I saw and felt in Don's brain was deadly, though, and I acted on impulse.

Don told me he was sending me an amethyst crystal—one that he had first lent me many years ago when I was having some elective surgery on my jaw. A picture of the crystal appeared on his audiotape *Crystal Meditations,* which I have played for nearly every guided imagery session I have ever led. Barbie Dossey told me she played the tape during her frequent bathe-and-relax rituals, and when it fell into the water after about ten years of use, she panicked. That's how good it is. Don rereleased the tape as part of his album called *Essence.*

Miriam and Harley Goldberg were present in many ways. As with the Dosseys, their contact, often daily during the bad old days, was itself pure medicine—medicine in the truest sense of "that which helps and heals." Harley is a physician who has trained himself in matters of body, mind, and spirit. Kaiser Permanente of northern California now has the good fortune to have him direct its alternative and complementary medicine section. Miriam is a psychotherapist and a dreamer, and I asked her to dream and image for me while I was intuitively incapacitated. Her dreams were detailed, mostly comforting, and often seemed to be a projection of my thoughts. Once or twice she appeared to be dreaming of medical options that I had known about but did not take, such as proton radiation done at the nuclear reactor. She dreamed of me in a wheelchair with a headpiece, which is what that treatment would have looked like. I did not like having anyone dream of me in a wheelchair, a highly undesirable possibility.

One dream sticks with me: Miriam saw me holding a whip as if in a circus, and everything around me was still. When I put down the whip, the action happened. I took that to mean that it was permissible to relinquish control and surrender to the circumstances—that it would be all right to do that for a change.

She was the first of many to have visions of me as a young girl, lying on a large bed, "quiet, not happy." Miriam said she was confused by this image and appearance and asked for more information. An eagle appeared (again, the eagle); walked around the child, nudging it with its beak; and placed jewels in the child's belly, throat, and forehead. "Much later," Miriam wrote, "an image of Jeanne connecting with eagle, and seeing and feeling the eagle in and as herself. This was a way to connect to the spirit world. She was radiant, in a boat, peaceful. Jeanne's throat was held in jewels. The sense was that when Jeanne connected to the spirit world via the eagle, she was then in good hands, so to speak." She saw the eagle again, and again it put jewels in my throat. Miriam actually gave me a carnelian, suggested in her dreams by the bird spirit, and I wore it on a thread around my neck.

Quickly I learned to put up my guard against projections and the New Age mentality. It wasn't as prevalent as one might suspect, but it was there from the get-go. "You need to ask yourself what you're afraid of seeing" was the most frequent bit of useless advice. Shit, there were plenty of things I didn't want to look at anymore, so I'd give them a list, which included the bank account and the dust mites under the bed, not to mention what was going on with my children, and it was usually more than anyone wanted to hear. No one who knew me well ventured onto this territory for long.

But here's the deal: There are things that you don't want to see, and it doesn't take a Ph.D. psychologist to figure this out and give it a name like "denial" or "dissociation" or whatever jargon is handy. But some things you just *can't* see, not if you look for months or years, because they are thickly disguised, twisted, or beyond the realm of conscious thought, and only in dreams and in the intuitive marrow of your bones do you know that "here be dragons," as the early mapmakers labeled uncharted and dangerous landscapes.

Daughter Lee Ann came down to Ventana from Monterey to spend the night and slept in one of our sleeping bags on the deck outside our room. She brought me marijuana, fine "bud," and told me how much it would help—a true gift of love, but unfortunately it doesn't work for me. She also brought insights. "The reason I sleep so much is that I imagine when I wake up next, I'll be able to see." Of course. Me, too. Chase stood us up for lunch—said his keys were locked in his truck. Maybe they were, or maybe he just couldn't face the family.

Before we left Ventana, we took doggie Yoshie's ashes and spread them around our old property and on his (and my) beloved Pfeiffer

Beach. The program director at Esalen Institute, Nancy Lunney, offered us space for four days in the beautiful VIP suite, situated at the edge of the cliffs, in full view of the air, water, and land that is nature's most majestic creation. Another dose of medicine, generously provided. Frank and I had massages every day and sat in the hot tubs under the stars at night. We saw friends, and I did some energy work with Vicki Topp, who gave me feedback that she felt "disconnections." "Something neuroendocrine. It feels like a soft, quiet depression."

Imagery and meditations were so unsatisfactory, blocked as they probably were by terror, so I decided to use a "Zen" paint set and draw. With this you dip a brush into water, draw on a board, and the image appears and then gradually disappears. I drew a fetus and then— almost with random strokes and with my nondominant hand—a graceful woman, a reclining, bent-over, sorrowing woman. Not only was she an appropriate image for how I felt, but the shape was identical to the image produced by the sonogram I would later have at the University of California at San Francisco.

Hours were spent in the meditation center, doing whatever I could to appease the clamor in my mind, and sitting on the cliffs overlooking the ocean that used to be my view and in the gardens where for years I had studied the plants and their habitat and recreated them as best I could, even in Santa Fe. The time was healing something.

———◇———

Frank and I then drove north, stopping by Chase's digs—a health hazard complete with a gas leak and a perpetual ooze from the shower pan—and took him a hamburger and grocery money (or at least that's what we told him to use it for).

"There's nothing wrong with you, Mom. You're going to be OK," he says, as he wolfs down the sandwich. Right. He and Frank have the same attitude. As for me, I'm about to throw up on the scrappy patch of weeds by Chase's front door. But maybe if he's hungry, he's OK. What do I know? But I can hope. He looks pretty good, actually, but says he still hasn't found the keys to his truck.

"I'll do anything you want me to."

"Get a job. That would help."

"OK. I'll get a job. I'll go looking for one tomorrow."

Whenever I see Chase or think about him, I feel like doubling over, disappearing, screaming, running away forever, dying, holding him, burning down the horrible place where he lives, shooting the face off every drug dealer in the world, taking him home, feeding him, trying one more time to bring this precious human back to life.

On to Melinda Maxfield's. Thank God for Mo and her estate, where, after this trip, as usual, she made me feel as though I'd reached Mecca. When you are in crisis at Mo's, you sit perched on the high stools in her kitchen. Friends, tea, schnapps, and chocolate appear miraculously, and the vigil is kept until it is no longer necessary, or when it is over, it's over, as they say. What I learned from her and the other girlfriends is that healing takes its own sweet time, and when you are in the midst of it, you just hang with one another and pay attention to needs at every level. It was not unknown for Mo to bark orders, sending me and other misbegotten souls to the rose garden, a hot bath, or to do some dance or song out by the pool. You just never knew. She draws her healing knowledge from traditions all over the world and makes some of it up as she goes along.

The Big Hand

{August 11}

AFTER SETTLING INTO this home-away-from-home, and filling a little bag with paraphernalia suitable for a night or two sequestered in the hospital, I left for the dreaded appointment with an ocular melanoma specialist, who will be known as Good Doc from here on out. I have chosen not to give his name because I'm not sure he would want to be known as the physician of a wild woman who, whether he totally approved or not, made her own treatment decisions, which were not considered "standard of care." In plain language that means you've gone off the trail.

Both this Eye Thing and my fear level were manageable as long as I did not have to be confronted with the Medical System. Even death was acceptable if I could do it my own way. From this moment onward it was just really clear that it was the System that brought me to my knees.

I am in the Hell Realm (or is it just Purgatory? I forget all those levels of waiting for Judgment Day) and hoping that Good Doc will not concur with the diagnosis. He says, "There is nothing else it could be." Another nasty sonogram. The Thing is bigger, much bigger; it is an elephant, the Empire State Building right there in my eye. How is it that something that supposedly took ten years to grow, and is "almost benign" but not quite, could grossly enlarge in less than two weeks? Even given differences in equipment, this does not make sense. The only explanation I ever got for it was, "Sometimes they just do this."

My heart sinks. They send me to the waiting room. In these eye places you get moved around from room to room, and you can spend the better part of a morning or an afternoon migrating. Interesting ritual. Frank has just come in, his eyes a wee bit shiny. I have never seen him cry in twenty-five years, and I'm wondering whether this dab of moisture might be the essence of tears. "What's wrong?" I ask.

"I'm tired. Had a hard time finding a parking place." I guess I am reassured that he still thinks nothing is really terminally wrong.

Good Doc is a likable and quite serious man and clearly fastidious. If anyone is going to handle an eye with skill and tenderness, it is he. When I first walked in his door, he said, "You have no idea how many people have already called me today to tell me you were coming in. You have so many who care for you."

What he can do, he says, is a "plaque" treatment. My tumor is on the edge of being too large, but he'll "go on a hunting expedition," he says.

"You trust me to do aggressive healing, and I will trust you with aggressive treatment," say I.

At this point I was desperate and would have gone for anything, short of eye removal. He, like all the others before and after, recommended poking my eye out as the first line of treatment. It is a strange litany that seems to be required before other suggestions are proffered.

What I soon learned from digging around in the medical literature is that enucleation (eye removal) is statistically likely to be followed by metastasis and death within weeks or months (the so-called Zimmerman effect). This information is based on a twenty-year-old study, and most ophthalmologists regard it as no longer being of consequence. They don't give any good reasons for disregarding the information except that the study is old. Spread of cancer following surgery has been reported with other types of cancer, and whether it is because the body is compromised from the trauma of anesthesia and surgery or whether "the knife" spreads disease is just speculation. There is growing evidence that an intact body fends off disease and that some tumors, not all, develop certain markers that trigger immune responses. If you take away the organ with the markers, or traumatize the body with too much surgery, the immune system loses its vanguard.

Surgery is a cure for many types of cancer, and I don't want to get into this argument, but let's use some sense here. Radical mastectomies, mutilative breast amputation down to the bone, have saved no more lives than lumpectomies, which are considerably gentler and more sparing of the body and the psyche.

Even though no one much believes (or will admit to believing) the eye-removal-followed-by-death information, several studies were conducted to see whether using radiation after the eye was removed decreased metastasis and increased survival. Obviously removing an eye was an unsatisfactory treatment, or they wouldn't have investigated the slash-and-burn technique. I don't want to even consider the gruesome and traumatic effects this procedure has on a face—especially what it would do to mine. Guess what? Poking it out and burning it don't guarantee a happy camper or a healthy one.

The plaque technique for ocular melanoma essentially involves sewing a bottle-cap–looking thing with radioactive pellets in it onto the back of your eye under general anesthesia, leaving it in place for five to seven days (while you yourself are radioactive and not allowed within six feet of human beings), and then removing it under general anesthesia. Two major surgeries. The results sounded pretty darn good: most of the time the tumor is burned out, which counts as "local control." In retrospect I have a few opinions about all this that I did not have in the beginning because I was in patient shock mode, as may clearly be surmised by this time. Many people are alive and well after the plaque treatment. Some even have a little vision return. I am happy for them and figure it is a rather effective treatment for tumors smaller than my Thing.

If you check on the Internet, you'll find proprietary Web sites that recommend places where you can get this procedure performed. Not too long ago, several treatment centers participated in a clinical trial for this technique, and now they are open for business and looking for customers, of which there will be few if this condition is as rare as they say.

Other people with large tumors who have the plaque treatment do ultimately go blind from glaucoma but may stay alive. Unfortunately I had this Godzilla thing in my eye, growing larger by the day, which is a pretty creepy thought in and of itself. I got to thinking, surgery that removes the eyeball in a manner of speaking and involves sewing in a shield embedded with radioactive materials would probably be pretty hard on a normal eye, much less one that seems a little incapacitated. Do I think a normal eye would survive the treatment? Hum. No one knows, and no one dares to ask or research this proposition. What idiot would allow this process on a normal eye? Nor am I excited about the prospect of two surgeries, two general anesthesias within a week. It has been my experience that this is not good for me, and in fact, I knew at some gut level that I could not survive the drugs. Whenever I mentioned my touchy history involving the near–body-bag experience and anesthesias and my Rasputinlike response to drugs, the response was inevitably, "You can talk to the anesthesiologist right before the surgery." No, no, they don't understand. This was serious business, and if they would just sit still long enough and listen, they might decide not to risk my life with two surgeries.

I wasn't sure whether I had made the choice for life as opposed to death just yet, but I did know my biochemistry was so bungled, I was so poisoned, that general anesthesia would not be survivable. I didn't want to go out that way, and to agree to it would have been suicide. I remember an old-time doctor who said he always asked his patients on the day of their surgery whether they thought it was a good day for it, and if they said "no," he'd learned the hard way that the procedure should be postponed until they gave an unqualified "yes."

So, anyway, Good Doc schedules me for next Tuesday, and I am as ready as I'll ever be. "Is there anything I can do to help myself in the meantime?"

"No."

"Is there anything I can do to avoid hurting myself?"

"Don't get hit on the head."

"By the way, what causes this thing?"

"Life." He's right.

Frank and I decided to drive home to Santa Fe on Thursday, and then I would fly back to California on Monday. I wanted to accompany him on the long trip across the country, and we did enjoy the pleasure of each other's company on the road. These were rare reflective times, driving across America, bad motels, scary food, and all.

Even though we had previously planned a two-week vacation with the Dosseys, Frank's anxiety level always rose each day he was separated from whatever business he had cooking. I didn't need that and neither did he, and besides, no one can come within six feet of a plaqued person, much less sleep in the same room. He might as well stay home.

Mo and Judy Ostrow were going to be my surgery pals. Both said they would take me to the hospital and stay there until I was ready to go home. We planned a party during the radioactive affair. Even Carl Simonton said he might join us. This time I left drawers full of clothes and all my toys (paints, books, and computer) in the upstairs bedroom at Mo's—as well as several attractive gowns suitable for convalescent salons, where I would sit at a distance.

Here's where the plot thickens and I begin to wonder, "Who is writing the script?" Two days later, on Friday the thirteenth, I called my answering machine from Laughlin, Nevada, where we spent the night, and I got little pleasure even from the nickel machines, my very favorite form of distraction. Hard to keep your mind on gambling under the circumstances. Turns out Dr. Good Doc's office was desperately trying to get in touch with me. "Geez," I think. "What now?" After careful consideration he has canceled the surgery and referred me to another doctor, who has "alternatives," meaning the nuclear reactor, otherwise known by me as "the bomb." Goody. I don't know why he changed his mind. Maybe because of the size of the monster he thought the alternative might be better.

For whatever reason I got derailed and referred one more time. Four eye docs in less than two weeks, and this was just the beginning.

Tomorrow would be the day to see whether I could get my head past the hell of medical treatment decisions, the Grim Reaper diagnosis, and follow my own advice and move into a bigger story, the metaphor. The medicine road had been a sinkhole into fear and despair. I was going under fast, feeling smaller and more insignificant by the minute.

Whew! We're only up to mid-August. These must be the longest days in history. I've got to change my outlook. Miracles really are happening in spite of everything, and they need to be recorded, if only to counterbalance the shit.

Son Chase says he has a job waiting tables at a restaurant in his neighborhood. He hasn't worked for a long time, and his dad and I quit sending him money when he dropped out of school in April. Lee Ann called when we got home. Her voice, sounding so strong, makes my heart sing.

Margaret Christensen and her friend Barbara, a psychotherapist, called. They told me of the prayer circle they had organized for me in Dallas and reminded me of the fact that I was living into a "bigger picture" and that my situation had major implications for so many people. Especially they talked about the relationship of my life to other women and to their children. Both have been touched by the Kosovars and saw my experience there as part of this larger story for women and their children.

How often I have told people that once the story of their lives had unfolded and some meaning was attached to the tragedy of illness, then healing, in the greater sense, could begin. These two women, on this day, nudged me past the immediacy of a terrible diagnosis and into the beginnings of that story. I cried for a long time after hanging up the phone, as I often did when compassion beyond measure was extended.

Margaret must be the most beloved ob-gyn in Dallas and surrounding territories. She gives her patients foot massages during labor and brought her own babies to her office, nursing them regardless of what else was going on. On her wall is a poster: "It pays to suck up to the boss." She practices medicine the way women should. Margaret has been in quite a few of my seminars and now conducts her own on women and healing. I knew from others that she was grief-stricken at hearing of my diagnosis and that she helped to carry on the Colorado workshop for women physicians after I bailed out suddenly right after the Grim Reaper diagnosis. I sent her my slides of women, and she told the story of women healers from ancient to modern times, which is what I had been scheduled to do for those days.

We're still on miracles here. Once in a while Frank and I start the day by drawing a tarot card and using the image to help focus our intentions. This morning Frank draws the Princess of Cups. In Angie Arrien's book of interpretations, this card advises one to be honest and to tell the truth. He is and does—especially about his own fears. He doesn't go into great detail about what his fears are, just that he is worried. That may not seem like a revelation, but it is the first time he's said he was concerned, and it's a big deal to me. Actually I'm glad he fooled me, covered up, and acted the stoic until now. Hysterics on the home front would only have complicated matters.

"How is Frank?" so many would inquire.

"I really don't know. He won't say much. Why don't you call him? He could use some attention and support."

Who called Frank, whom he called back, what was said, I don't know. His maintenance attitude toward what was happening to me was that there was just no problem—period. Everything was fine. It was a misdiagnosis. Only once did I detect some second thoughts, and that was after he had a conversation with a psychiatrist with whom he worked who had done her residency at Massachusetts Eye and Ear, probably the best-known treatment center in the country for these diseases.

No more than a day later, he told me he had found a physician who said that I should be able to have all the drugs I wanted and was willing to prescribe them for me. Who the physician was or what this implied, I do not know. Was it for Plan B? Or in case the whole business got too grisly and painful? The questions remained unasked because Frank most likely would not have answered them, and besides, just now I was fine, thank you very much. With the single exception of mentioning my situation to two oncologists with whom he worked, this was the only active recommendation or information Frank ever brought home. Drugs. I would certainly keep this idea in mind. They might be useful someday.

A woman who must remain nameless called with good news. She had been doing radionics for me for the past two weeks. This is a system of "energy healing" using machines. Judy Ostrow had insisted on it, telling me it had helped her avoid several things, perhaps even including breast cancer. Judy has had several suspicious lumps, which were found to be harmless, much to the amazement of her physicians. When Judy and the other girls tell me to do something, I usually do, even if I don't believe in it. Some of the time they are right. At the very least, I figure the radionics machine is a tool, like a dowsing rod, that reflects the invisible world of the intuition. The inner knowing is always present; we just don't always know how to access it and bring it into conscious awareness.

As a treatment methodology, radionics strains my belief system; as a tool for mining the intuition, it does not. I've been proceeding intuitively anyhow, flying by the seat of my pants, so I might as well get a better understanding of how this intuition business works.

The radionics machines need some part of you—spit, skin, whatever—to make the diagnosis. When working at a distance, you are asked to send hair that has not been chemically treated. Now, I ask you, how many of us have untreated hair on our heads? The FedEx envelope containing a rather large sample of my pubic hair was misdelivered twice, and I had the fleeting thought that if it had been opened accidentally, I could well have become a legend in my own time.

The woman validated the diagnosis of ocular melanoma. I had an original tumor load of four hundred and something, whatever that means. Today she said the mass was 65 percent blood and most of the rest some kind of fibrous material. She named a few toxins in my eye. The only problem with this was that, over time, virtually every substance imaginable was found in my eye: fungi, parasites, chemicals, and viruses. Could be, I suppose. Maybe, as the dream in Macedonia said, that is my "sponge," the repository of all the poisons of my life.

◇

I was still focused on miracles the following day. I got out *Spontaneous Remission,* by Brendan O'Regan and Caryle Hirshberg. The book had been in the oven for about fifteen years before it was published. I felt a part of it only because Brendan was the research director at the Institute of Noetic Sciences and he and I had spent days together in Fort Worth and San Francisco. He escorted me on my first tour of San Francisco, thereby initiating my lifelong love affair with the city. The institute gave its first grant to Carl and Stephanie Simonton for research on the mind-body aspects of cancer. The money came from a donated car—a Mercedes, if I remember correctly. Most of it went to pay my salary as researcher for the Simontons' work. In this book I read for the first time about spontaneous remissions of ocular melanoma. Given the rarity of this particular cancer, quite a few remissions have been reported. In fact, it appeared to be one of the tumors more likely to go into remission.

Today I also worked in my magnificent gardens. They are full of psychedelic-hued flowers, aromatic herbs, and enough vegetables to feed us for months. The hollyhocks are six feet high. As a matter of fact, almost everything is taller than I am. The sweet peas and morning glories had finally covered the tepee in the middle of the cut-flower and vegetable garden. While working in the dirt, I remembered a dream from last summer—who could forget it?—that I was struck by lightning while mulching the rows by the gate.

Today, too, I found healing and solace in the sauna and in the room where I keep my holy things—both dark places.

I read Robbie Gass's book *Chanting* and adopted his mantra, "I choose life." Robbie later told me that it was more than a mantra. He would sit in his meditation places and say it over and over, and all sorts of reasons would come up about why he was not choosing life or why he didn't want to live. He also said the mantra when he walked, all the time, everyplace.

It was a long day.

The Medicine Dance Begins

{August 16}

I GOT UPGRADED to first class on the way to California. Another miracle, because almost all the travelers, like me, have a million miles on their records. I didn't know when I'd return or in what condition, but I had what I needed stored at Mo's for the duration.

Mara Jan Bradbury (another girlfriend who qualifies as a miracle in the annals of health caring) met me at the airport. I call her the "Road Warrior." She drives up and down the California coast in her well-stocked Range Rover; she drives when she's unnerved, when she's happy, when she needs to help someone. Sometimes she bolts out in the middle of the night and drives five hundred miles. From the airport we went to the Eye Place. Now I'm going to get really vague. The exact names and places are not important. It's easy to take a cheap shot at medicine right now, and I don't want to be among the bombardiers. The events related to my treatment (and lack thereof) could have happened anywhere.

As Mara Jan said later, the Eye Place was in the Twilight Zone. We might try to find it again, only to discover that it had disappeared from the face of the earth. Maybe we were never there. The city had been in one of its dark moods all summer and was gray and cold, and so was the Eye Place. We were the only human forms of life when we got there. There was hand-lettered signage relating to its affiliated institutions. Hand lettering does not inspire confidence.

Mara Jan parked me in some desolate waiting area and went back to the car to get us more clothes because we were freezing to death. She seemed to have quite a selection of sweaters and jackets, and I was glad, as usual, that I would not be in uncoordinated attire even in adverse circumstances. She also brought in almonds, which she fed me periodically "to keep my energy up." We stood right outside the doctor's office and used Mara Jan's cellular phone to call the answering machine and let whoever wasn't there know we had arrived. A few people finally drifted in, since it was the end of the lunch hour. No one looked up to help us until we made grunting and snorting noises that simply could not be ignored.

The Eye Doc is present, honest, and kind. A story is told about an experience with E.D.'s father. The physician at some treatment facility had said there was no hope and refused to do treatment. "Go home and die." (Boy, I've heard that one a few times.) E.D. spirits Pop out of the treatment center to another one that is more positive and offers some therapy. Pop is still alive after nine years. E.D. is obviously familiar with the mind-body connection, and when I ask what I can do, I am told, "Just think positive." I wonder whether E.D. knows that this is my line.

The medical nightmare continues, though. The yarn is being spun. My diagnosis is obviously a done deal before I get in the door.

These specialists in ocular melanoma claim to make no mistakes, or few, in diagnosis. Some published studies say that the diagnoses are 97 to 99 percent accurate by visual inspection. In other words, the specialists can tell what the problem is just by looking in the eye. They also write about how often problems that are initially diagnosed as being attributable to other conditions really turn out to be melanoma. Never the opposite is true. False negatives but no false positives to speak of. You have to wonder, though, whether they ever snag out an eye and then say, "Whoops, we made a little mistake here." If they do, they don't write about it.

The E.D.'s fingers are strong and efficient as equipment is adjusted and drawings of the images of the sprawling Thing are made in my chart. I note how dark everything is. All these eye places are dark, but I guess if you want to see into someone's soul, you need to turn off the lights. I am the only patient of the day, and we spend three hours going from one room to the next. Mara Jan has brought in a tape recorder, but for various reasons, we do not get the session taped. The closet anthropologist in me wonders whether this is a sacred event, and if so, it is not to be recorded except in memory. I had three pages of questions that Mara Jan and I went over while she drove to the city. At the end of our time with E.D., I feel that my questions have been answered, but they really were not—a fact that neither Mara Jan nor I realized until after we left.

The treatment under consideration for me now was proton radiation, and I was informed it was noted for precision, because the rays could "bend" and thereby avoid damaging healthy tissue. I asked about the destruction that proton radiation might cause to a normal eye. Vague answer. These were not trick questions—I really wanted to know. The eye is a very tiny, sensitive area. I wanted to know because, if I decided to go through with this, I planned on living for a while, and I didn't want to be made sicker by the treatment, nor did I want my face to fall off. Anyway, I had a clue about radiation. I had worked as a technical assistant in the Department of Radiation Biology at Texas A&M for a year as an undergraduate and watched the effects of very small doses of radiation on goats and rats. Not good.

"How many people have you treated with this diagnosis?" "Oh, lots of them. I've had several referred this week." Not the correct answer, but in my stunned-out-of-my-gourd state, I do not probe. I wanted to know how many people with this diagnosis had been treated at this particular nuclear reactor and what the results were. This information had to be available. It would be the skills of the radiation oncologist that would determine the accuracy of the radiation, and who that individual would be wasn't revealed. The E.D.'s role was merely to sew in a protective shield behind the eye, and although I was asking the right questions, I was apparently directing them to the wrong person.

"What is the effect of no treatment?" was a question that never got asked because it was very clear from the conversation that not treating the condition would mean progressive disease and death, and even to ask it would be heresy. Watch and wait was not going to be an option with this bad boy in my eye. "How can you plan treatment on a mass that has changed shape fairly constantly over the past few weeks? How can you be sure of hitting the target?" Again, I was asking the wrong question or the wrong person.

"What color is the tumor?" I ask this because it helps my imagery. "Brownish. But they don't have to be brown, you know. I have even seen white ones." So the tumor has changed color, along with practically every other characteristic, in less than three weeks. Lively little devil.

"Do you think you can do radiation on it?" E.D. shrugs and says it depends on the oncologist's decision. This is the first mention of an oncologist. I am naive. I ask about the immune properties. I've been reading that melanomas are very sensitive to immune stimulation.

"Yes, but the eye down-regulates when faced with an antigen. It is counterintuitive."

"It does what?"

"The eye doesn't like to be inflamed. So instead of up-regulating, it down-regulates. There are only a few people in the world who know much about eye immunology. It is a system unto itself."

So here we go. The Queen of Psychoneuroimmunology has an immune problem that does not follow the rules. I can't believe it. Normally foreign bodies, viruses, bacteria, or cancer cells, known collectively as antigens, incite the immune system to attack. The defense involves inflammation, or heat and swelling, from the activity of immune cells and chemicals. The eye can't afford to have too much immune activity because it might destroy delicate structures. Later I found out it was not quite so simple: the eye does experience inflammatory activity during darkness, but when it is exposed to light, the inflammatory activity decreases.

I wrote in my journal that this E.D. was "OK, but I have the feeling that I will still have major challenges in the medical system." (That was an understatement.) I am still desperate to have the Thing gone. Now I am afraid that it has gotten too big to treat even with the bomb. I am ready to beg and scuttle to have my eye burned out.

The tests that follow are abusive. Another sonogram. The image of the growth looks just like a fetus. Mara Jan and the lab tech (who is friendly and obviously knows her work) gasp as the fetal form emerges on the screen.

The lab tech says, "You're fortunate."

"Why?"

"It's only this big," and she points to a millimeter scale.

"Have you seen larger ones?"

"Oh, much." First time anyone has acted as if it weren't the size of Mars. I ask her why the tumor seemed to lack mass on the ultrasound. Again, I get an answer that is a nonanswer but don't realize it at the time. She says, "That's how you diagnosis a primary ocular melanoma." Somewhat relieved, I shut up. Primary is better than secondary, which would mean it was a metastasis from some other site and would make the prognosis even worse.

More pictures of the back of my eyes. And—the worst of all—an orange dye is injected into my artery so that the blood pattern in my eye can be photographed. "It's just a vegetable dye," the guy says, a syringe about ten inches long, if memory serves me correctly, poised to plunge. I don't recall reading any informed consent on this procedure, but there should have been, and I'm not wild about this much orange anything being shot into an artery. I turned orange immediately. My bathwater that night was orange, and I peed orange juice. It also gave me a migraine that made me crazy and cross-eyed, on one of the days when I was on an airplane trying to get home. Whenever I've mentioned this since, the comment has been, "We'll make a note in your chart." When and if the time comes, I hope someone reads that chart, because it's certainly supposed to contain quite a few notes.

When the sonogram is finished, E.D. looks in the door. I am fully aware that I have taken up far too much time and pressed the system beyond its limits, and know that I am likely to get blasted into silence, but there are still some questions. It is my eye, my life, and I ain't done yet with data collection. I ask whether there were any surprises from the tests.

"No, there were not. I will try to bump you up in the waiting line for the nuclear reactor."

The facility is used for medical purposes only about two days a month, so treatment has to be carefully orchestrated. Before the radiation, though, a shield will first be sewn behind my eye and allowed to heal for about a week. There is a specified time period for healing, and allowing too much time or not enough is not optimal.

Major surgery. The good news is, I can spend the night across the street from the surgery unit in another hospital where the people aren't so sick, and I can still be watched for pain control. I'm beginning to get the picture: I'll initially be treated in an awful place, then moved to one that is less so, and this procedure is not going to be exactly painless.

What I Need Now

{August 17}

BACK TO MIRACLES. At Mo's house the girlfriends convene. Mara Jan disappears while Mo and I ramble on about our usual topics, and then she magically reappears with fresh corn on the cob and ripe tomatoes from a nearby farm. Angie Arrien does a check-in call and tells me the "Cyclops" myth. Cyclops sacrificed an eye so he could see the truth, both inside and outside. Then Angie relates the four tasks of the next phase of the feminine, and I am touched. They are (1) defining the feminine, (2) knowing true self, (3) bonding with the sisterhood, and (4) awakening the world. Makes me tired to think of these challenges, but she's absolutely correct, of course.

I found notes in my journal that I must have written on the airplane home:

What I Need and Don't Need

1. Talk to no one who wants to connect with me so they will feel better.
2. Avoid language of "beat this," "fight," or people who need me as a warrior icon.
3. Release into the process—the fullness of the human condition—gather wisdom to help light the world—turn inward and look—protect myself.
4. Heal motherhood issues by teaching my children to care.

5. Stay awake—stay clear, trust body, trust life, soften what has hardened.
6. Open what has been closed.
7. Remember the "awesome beauty and terror," the "exhilaration of being on the edge of being" (from Anatole Broyard, *Intoxicated by My Illness*).

For imagery I wrote that I could imagine that the DNA needs to be uncoupled and the chain realigned, and I imaged wriggling snakes, my body mounting an inflammatory response. I could help it by detoxing, eating live food, and changing the way I think about things, not necessarily in that order.

I also wrote that I need to carry my own light with my pride, that I should cancel things, turn off, and try to stay focused inward. I had exhausted my font of talent, vision, and creativity. I wrote that I needed to quit teaching for some time. Some teachers seem to be able to give the same lecture for a lifetime. I can't. I get bored. My ideas change faster than my lecture notes, and when slides turn brownish, I've used them too long.

In the creative wasteland of the last six years, I have been stripped of my ideas and questioned my dogma. If I must teach (and that seems to be my task), what now? I ask, again, Where is my mentor on the Other Side, Ginny Hine, in this process? I have been too long the focus of projections and needs that do not belong to me. I need to make daily life a ritual, gather wisdom. Then my vision will return. I draw an eye and a heart.

Turnaround Time

{August 18}

THE DAY TO END ALL. A "turnaround." It begins with absolutely the crowning misery of my personal experience of the modern profession of medicine—the lack of caring for people who are in crisis and the senselessness of an inhumane system. Notice that I am not complaining about the doctors but about the system, and the extent to which they are responsible for it is a matter of debate.

The morning starts with a call from someone I don't know who tells me that I have been scheduled for an appointment on September 1 with a radiation oncologist about two thousand miles away. I'm told, not asked. So I call the Eye Doc's office and find out that I've been scheduled for surgery less than a week from this very day—again, a couple of thousand miles away—and for radiation four weeks later and the radiation oncologist somewhere in between.

The medical system strikes fear into the hearts of the bravest, and that's certainly what it did to me. This is very bad medicine, regardless of intentions. The metal-shield surgery was going to be performed before the radiation oncologist had given the go-ahead to do radiation. Sewing a metal shield behind an eye is serious business and highly unlikely to be beneficial per se. What if the radiation oncologist subsequently said the tumor was too large for radiation and I'm stuck with the trauma from the surgery? All the eye people I had seen, including Good Doc and the Eye Man, had suggested that the Thing might be too large for treatment. What if I really didn't have a melanoma and all this was done to an eye that might have had an infection or a bleed, as suggested by the MRI report, shoddy as it was?

One of the definitive tests, the orange dye job, had not yet been developed or its results read. None of the ophthalmologists had looked at my MRIs, which were equivocal. And I had been told that there was an optimum healing period between the metal-shield surgery and the radiation—about a week—and that too short or too long a healing period was not good. The interval in the proposed scenario would be more than three weeks. No, no, no. This felt all wrong, and I felt helpless and intimidated. I remember uncoordinated medical systems. There was a scandal at one hospital where I worked when two amputations were done on one guy because they cut off the wrong limb the first time. Nope. I need a medical system that can demonstrate it has its act together before anyone puts me under with modern chemistry and removes, adds, or manipulates anything.

Sandy Ingerman called when I was sitting at my desk, frozen and dispirited. She had just done a shamanic journey, and her spirits had told her that I must *not* do anything against my faith and belief. The spirits informed her there was some urgency about conveying this message, and it probably saved my life.

I stopped the medical process immediately, and was rescheduled for the next month. I asked that my records be sent for a second opinion from the Big Dogs of treatment for ocular melanoma. This should have been done earlier, but I had been far too overwhelmed with the daily activities of life, upon which was superimposed the possibility of Plan B for death, and I had not thought of everything. Never have a body part destroyed without a second or third opinion.

Then, around two o'clock, an interesting thing happened: the fear left my life and would not return until months later, when I had another encounter with the medical system. My body felt soft and my heart less cramped. My biochemistry changed. Was all that prayer finally kicking in? I was getting more and more calls about prayers and prayer circles, so maybe a critical mass of praying had been reached.

Larry LeShan called, reminding me to recapture the Western spiritual tradition—which in each soul is the seed of a flower. Our soul ("sole") task is to nurture it into bloom. He reminded me that I'd said I had lost my vision and that only if I recaptured it would the tumor regress. It was a great call, actually.

I also spoke with Barbie and Larry Dossey. I walked in blessings and beauty. These are all miracles. My intuition is that something turned on this complicated day.

I also made a note in my journal of pills and potions that I was doing serious detoxification—two saunas daily, megasupplements, and eating food from my organic garden, which meant mostly carrots, beans, and lettuce of many hues.

Frank and I were in Indiana on the weekend of August 19, teaching imagery and body-mind consciousness to a group of professionals who meet with us four times a year. These groups are about the most fun thing I do: the people are lively, engaged, and we come full circle as a family over the year, learning from one another.

I have an innate distrust of teachers who are not truthful (not that they have to tell the whole truth, but they shouldn't lie) or who act as if they've never been sick a day in their lives and it is somehow a moral transgression to be so. There are those on the speaking circuit who are chronically or mortally ill, hide it, and criticize illness as some character flaw. Not smart. Not clean. So I give the class the basics on my "challenge."

The participants are responsive and touched. As usually happens, the work has a broader implication: at least two others in the class have also received an unusual diagnosis and face the prospect of maiming treatment with no promise of a healthy outcome. The teaching is elevated far beyond the usual material because several are living the experiences.

During the weekend the shaman Michael Harner returned my call and offered to work with me. "Two nights would be good, but three better. I am pretty much free whenever you can come the whole month of September."

Good news, oh such wonderful news! Michael, an acquaintance of more than twenty years, is probably the best-known shaman in the Western world. He wrote *The Way of the Shaman* and has brought shamanism and the core teachings of shamanic practice back to cultures that have forgotten their own traditions, to shamans who still carry drums but have forgotten what they are for. I trust him with my life, and being able to experience his vast repertoire of access to the spirit world would bring some measure of virtue to this difficult healing process.

I was excited, exalted, high. Whoopee! I hung up the phone and ran to find Frank and tell him the fantastic news. He could go with me. Frank had engaged in shamanistic practices with a few of his patients, and what an opportunity this would be to expand his own skills, learn from a master teacher, and be present during such a precious time for me.

"Darling, I can't just take off work for these things. I have my own life to live."

"But you could come for the weekend, maybe?"

"No, no I can't. You don't have anything that is life-threatening, you know." That's what Frank said when I told him the news.

Months later Frank said that what he *meant* was, I was not in a life crisis at the time, which I suppose meant a situation that was imminently life-threatening, but it left me with permanent concerns about where I could find help if I needed it. I went into emotional gridlock because I had choices to make. I could fly like a lone eagle, but the fucking vision thing meant that I was, like it or not, temporarily impaired and would have to obtain services. For starters, I'd need to hire a car and a driver. The Fates forced me to ask for help, because if it had been any other part of my body needing care, if I could have seen where I was going, I would not have reached out as much as I did. So I called in the flock. Mo was going to be home on September 8–10, and she would be honored to drive, drum for the journey, and anchor the space or whatever. Mara Jan could be there also.

I am not writing about my feelings now, and I am remembering again those women's journals of the Wild West in which they noted their remarkable circumstances and not their emotions. Why bother? Words are too small, too wasted, and they only etch the pain in more deeply. Anyway, who with a human heart would not know how I was feeling?

After the training we picked up my daughter, Lee Ann, at the airport. I had a small window of time before traveling again, and I really wanted to have her come see me in Santa Fe. She had a dream that night that someone broke into our house, trashed several rooms, and broke one of the goddess statues. Actually one was broken—a ceramic woman, painted to look like a bronze, and holding a crystal ball. Lee Ann said she and I were trying to clean things up when she awoke.

––––––◇––––––

A prayer from Margaret Christensen came in the mail a couple of days later and brightened my life:

> Healer, Teacher, Mentor, Friend, Woman of Great Vision. Images
>   bring you in sight now, one eye sees outward into the Light
> Both worlds of immense beauty and profound devastation
> One eye sees inward into the Dark, waiting to unveil the wisdom
>   there.
> You have been chosen to look into the Void and be surrounded by it.
> To articulate for us the teachings there. Your gifts have helped many
>   on this journey, the time has come for you to walk it now.
> Surrounded in Love by those who hold your sacred space,
> Walking with courage and humility into the Fear
> You will not be lost for we will sing you home
> You feel those whom you have loved, touched, taught, healed.
> You sense friends, teachers, guides, and creatures that have mentored
>   you.
> Gathered around the darkness our healing prayers coalesce,
> An intense beam of Light enters your eye, illuminating the coal-black,
>   nebulous cloud.
> Experiences of dark, of fear, of pain, of evil, implode into a tiny
>   diamond-like prism. This crystal of Sight scintillates,
> Fear is transformed to power to clearly see the Truth.

Margaret and so many others reminded me that there are still healers in the profession of medicine, that I was not alone, and that they would sing me home.

Kill-or-Cure Routine

{August 23}

THIS MARKS THE BEGINNING of serious research on the kill-or-cure self-help routine—which eventually proved to be a mixture of whatever I could find that had any potential whatsoever to stimulate immune function. I forget whom all I called, but I was on the telephone for several days. One call led to another, and I scribbled notes all over my "Visions" journal.

The Internet information produced by searching on the keyword "eye" scared the shit out of me, and I have avoided Web searches assiduously ever since. Although the Web may be revolutionizing the consumer role in health care, I found the information available there just revolting, not only for my supposed diagnosis but for others, such as brain tumors, as well. Clinics, researchers, and clinicians are trolling for patients. The mortality and morbidity figures reported on these Web sites are alarmist and couched in language that is frightening. These are scare tactics. I didn't need them just now.

I spoke with Gar Hildebrand, a very good man who has been part of what I call the "cancer boy" community, which has doggedly tried to change the way cancer is treated. He sent me material about the Gerson cancer treatment, which he had researched for a long time, and initiated European connections. Following Gar's advice and the information he sent me, I brewed organic coffee for enemas and cooked up the "cancer stew," a mixture of mushed-up vegetables, eating it as often as possible. Neither the enemas nor the stew is really bad. It did take about three days to get the hang of the enemas, though, without spewing coffee all over the bathroom, on every towel and rug, and running down the walls. I called Fleur Green, a local girlfriend, because I knew she'd done a few herself or at least had friends who had done them. (We have been sisters under the skin, by the way, since the moment we met and discovered we frequented the same dress shop. We looked like brides-maids in our nearly identical clothes.)

Fleur said, "Just do it. You get so you like it. You have all that time alone, and nobody bothers you. Think of it like a thirty-minute medita-tion."

"What do you mean 'all that time'? It only takes three minutes." Obviously I had been rushing the process a little.

I tried two "coffee breaks" and two saunas a day, which takes up several hours. I tried to do imagery with the coffee breaks. Gar told me that they "race" bile turnover and liver enzymes and that helps clear the blood of toxins, so that's what I imagined. He and others began the international fact-seeking network for me. The clinics in Germany that specialize in immunotherapy sounded the most promising, but none of them had ever treated a primary ocular melanoma, as best we could determine. The director of the one with the best reputation re-fused to accept me as a patient until I had "that terrible tumor" treated—meaning, I guess, eye removal.

Ralph Moss, one of the leading and most respected proponents for taking new directions in cancer care, not only returned my calls but also gave me his telephone number at a vacation retreat. He prepared a file for me—very factual, no bullshit—and sent it to me gratis, although this is his business, called *The Moss Reports*. I am extremely grateful and don't expect such generosity. The report starts by reviewing standard medical information and then gives information about the alternatives, together with Ralph's astute opinion regarding those alternatives. I've known Ralph since we were both on a committee around 1988 for the Office of Technology Assessment, the research arm of Congress at that time. Our assignment was to study "unorthodox" cancer treatments. It was a zoo: people picketed; there was even a bomb threat, if I re-member correctly; and the passion for change was high. After all, cancer care is a matter of life and death. It was at that time that I got a true appreciation for the hard work done behind the scenes on cancer. It is because of Ralph, Senator Tom Harken, former representative Berkeley Bedell, Gar Hildebrand, and on and on, that cancer care and research might just move out of the dark ages. They are the real foundation for any changes in cancer care and were the stimulus for extraordinary movements within governmental funding, such as the National Institutes of Health's establishment of the National Center for Complementary and Alternative Medicine.

Ralph suggested that I contact Nick Gonzalez, M.D., in New York. Ralph and others feel that Nick has had some of the most successful treatment outcomes, and unlike many, Nick has kept good records. Because his work is so careful and promising, the National Cancer Institute is funding a five-year study of his work—a milestone for alternative therapies. The study made headlines in the health section of the *New York Times*. I am glad for him.

"He may be hard to reach," Ralph said, "and sometimes he just refuses to take people as patients, especially if they are evading the traditional medical system."

Nick turned out to be very accessible and informative, and he made no judgment on whether I was evading the medical system, which I sort of was and sort of wasn't. I am reminded why the world of alternative medicine has retained such a hold on my own life: it is not only full of promise but full of heart. I don't know enough words to use to thank these people. Everyone I talked to went way beyond the call of duty. Many phone periodically just to see how I'm feeling. I've often been told, "Just ask. We'll do anything we can for you." And then they say something about how grateful they are for my long dedication to the field of cancer. When I hear this, I am not so sure my work has made an important enough contribution to warrant such praise or kindness. But thanks, anyway.

I'm convinced both that Nick's program is effective and that it must become a lifestyle. You need to do the entire process, not just a thing or two here and there. No cheating. Nick prescribes special diets, which may even include meat; coffee enemas; enzymes and supplements up the wazoo. I decided that I could not do the program just now—or rather, I chose not to do it just now—because it is very arduous. I keep it tucked away in the back of my mind, "if and when."

After reading the research, though, I did decide to order similar enzymes and stuff them down. Some you're even supposed to take in the middle of the night, which was just fine because I was up most of the night anyway. The explanation that supports gagging down all these pills is that tumors develop a protein coat that protects them from identification and attack by the immune system. The enzymes digest that protein. As we get older, our own enzymes get sluggish and need some help. The major side effect is that your body secretions reek of tomcat piss.

Ed Tyska, a well-informed doctor friend of many years, recommended (and sent) a huge carton of supplements, including maitake mushrooms, thymus gland pills, and Cellular Forté (a supplement that is supposed to stimulate natural killer cell activity). I take it all. He emphasizes, almost as a mantra, "Remember, you are not your body. There is more."

Life goes on. I do not feel particularly well, but to this day, I can't separate out fear from disease from the effects of putting so many immune stimulants into my body or from stress. With so much going on, one turns into a seething chemical stew.

Nothing happens with the eye, except maybe more loss of vision. I am looking forward to Michael Harner's work and planning on going to England on September 19 with Judy to teach and to be with Jean Sayre-Adams and Steve Wright. Why not? I've heard nothing from the E.D.'s office either, so I can repress any nasty thoughts of medical treatment for a little while longer.

Lee Ann is still in Santa Fe, but she sleeps all day, I've discovered. She prowls around at night, which must have something of a genetic basis. We had a full moon, so she even planted some irises after midnight. I think she's making great progress. She runs up and down our hill, works in the garden, seems to have energy and enthusiasm, just at odd times. She sits and looks at the TV even though her vision is such that she can't see all colors and her acuity is limited. She also smokes constantly, but I have absolutely given up worrying about such things. It's her life.

Someone from my Indiana workshop sent me this poem by Dawna Markova. It gets placed on my refrigerator and becomes my creed:

I will not die an unlived life.
I will not live in fear
Of falling or catching on fire.
I choose to inhabit my days
To allow my living to open me,
To make me less afraid,
More accessible,
To loosen my heart
Until it becomes a wing,
A torch, a promise.
I choose to risk my significance,
To Live
So that which came to me as seed goes to the next as blossom
And that which came to me as blossom, goes on as fruit.

Mistletoe and Dreams

{August 27}

AN E-MAIL IS CIRCULATED for my healing, which I suspect was initiated by Crystal Hawk, a Canadian friend who has a worldwide network of Therapeutic Touch practitioners. Therapeutic Touch is a non-contact method of energy healing used by many people, most of them nurses, in medical settings all over the world. I had hesitated until this time to ask for any healing web or networking attention because I didn't want to wear people out over my cause and because the diagnosis still just didn't feel correct to me. By late August, more than a month after the diagnosis and still no treatment plan in sight, Crystal asked me what I needed. I was aware of how badly I needed support. I couldn't have felt much worse than I did then. So many people were asking for information, so I wrote:

> I am still in the unknown. The thing will probably be irradiated—but we need to finish tests, etc. I am feeling the need to be held in the light of love and trust and healing energy. This is really the "acute" period of chaos. Once there is a plan, I can deal with it. This is challenging every aspect of my being. I need some long-distance Therapeutic Touch. Please do a healing web as soon as possible.
>
> Love,
> Jeanne

Responses came from everywhere, as far away as New Zealand. I was placed on many prayer lists and prayer circles, and Crystal forwarded me many of the responses from old friends and people who knew me through my writing and presentations, and from others who respond when they are called upon to pray, no matter whom it is for.

The following day marked the beginning of many important communications from Steve Wright, with whom I learned to feel a bond of lifetimes: "I got the news today and felt numb. I will not bother you with platitudes. Please know that you are in my prayers and thoughts with loving concern and wishes for your well-being. I am so glad you will be with us in September."

By now I had decided that going to England was more vital to my healing than staying home and being doctored, cut, burned, or whatever was in store for me.

From Jeannie Sayre-Adams, Steve's partner and my friend: "I had a healing dream about you early this morning. We were in an airplane, and the healing had begun."

Jeannie and Steve are nurses and healers, teach Therapeutic Touch and other forms of healing, and I trust their intuitions. These messages gave me courage and bolstered my belief that healing was possible.

About this time I get the idea that I need to use mistletoe. I am not sure how this decision was made—maybe reading, listening, and hearing Carl Simonton say that it is part of the standard of care in many hospitals in Germany. It is used by a system of medicine called anthroposophy, which I respect very much. It was founded by Rudolf Steiner, whose work is best known in the United States from the Waldorf schools.

Mistletoe fits well into my belief system. A sacred plant from the Celts and before, mistletoe represents the end of the old Nordic order, the twilight of the gods. How perfect for me, Jeanne the Viking Queen.

The medicine is grown on different host trees, such as oak (*Quercus*) and apple, and is harvested and prepared with precision. As with all Steiner-based horticulture, it is grown within an organic system that attends to the broad ecological environment. Mistletoe is brought into this country in injectable ampoules as a legal homeopathic remedy, but it is not highly diluted the way most homeopathics are.

The anthroposophic doctors are M.D.'s, but their practice of medicine has a deeply interwoven spiritual thread. I visited one of their cancer hospitals in Freiburg, Germany, a few years ago and, jaded though I may be, was impressed with the whole healing scene—music, sculpture therapy, massage with aromatic oils, good medicine, and respect for the healing arts and the patients who were receiving treatment. Anthroposophy is the only modern system of healing that has emerged out of a metaphysical or spiritual basis, came from a Western basis of thought, and includes allopathic (conventional) medicine when appropriate. Other living systems of healing, such as Tibetan medicine and Ayurvedic medicine, evolved much earlier and from cultural roots of the Eastern traditions.

I called the manufacturing company myself and spoke with a doctor. He consulted other colleagues in Switzerland, and they decided that Quercus Series I would be appropriate for me, so a physician who was working with my "case" (don't we all love being called "cases"?) prescribed it for me. There are several in the series for each tree, and Series I was of medium strength. Quercus is usually prescribed for men, not women. I didn't question this, because I had put myself on a path in which I had to trust the unusual and not do so much arguing.

The research on mistletoe as an immune stimulant is superb. The plant is intelligent. It kills tumors *and* increases immune function, which is highly unusual in a single substance. The research has been done on humans in clinical trials, on animals, and in cultures outside the body. In treatment of humans, a mood elevation is usually noted, as well as return of appetite and energy, which is why it is used as an adjunct to other treatment. For these reasons alone, mistletoe is a useful therapy.

About once a year or so, Carl and I talk about the classic Krebiozen story. Krebiozen was a supposedly worthless drug used for cancer treatment, but while it was being tested, it got some good press. One guy with lung cancer took it, and within days his "tumors melted like snowballs on a hot stove." Then Krebiozen got some bad press. The tumors came back. No one could ethically pull this off now, but his doctors decided to give him a saline injection and tell him it was Krebiozen (a more potent batch); the tumors disappeared almost before their very eyes. The patient died quickly, though, when the drug made headlines again as absofuckinlutely worthless. Mistletoe may be my own form of belief-medicine, as Krebiozen was to many others.

Only a handful of physicians use mistletoe in the United States, and mostly for HIV. All the research has been done in Europe, but the results have been published in English, so there is no excuse for not being aware of it. The researchers and clinicians are all very careful not to tout mistletoe as a cure but instead present it as a supportive treatment for use in conjunction with radiation, surgery, or immunotherapy. Matter of fact, I know of no other preparation that is so versatile and powerful and yet does no damage to intact cellular structures. When mistletoe is shot into the primary tumor, superior results are reported. I'd almost have been willing to have that done, but the mistletoe eventually gravitated toward my eye on its own, so I guess it knew where to go.

———◇———

I dance, not too gracefully, between one level of healing and the next. An E-mail comes from Steve Wright on the last day of August to remind me that the transpersonal realm of healing is much more important to me than the biological one:

> Unbeknownst or not, Jeannie and I have been working with you. There is some hesitation about sending you this message because I still, after all this time, lack confidence in these things. Also you must be getting lots of help, and I don't want to confuse you. But Jeannie says I must, sooooooo . . .

> 1. I'm sending you some help in several tangible forms, in the post, this morning. The first is a string of beads bought at Mother Meera's and held onto for a long time, with the thought that someday someone would need these. I had visitors last week. I was showing them around the house. When we got to my studio, their delightful, brilliant, shiny child made a beeline for my altar. For some reason I wasn't worried as he launched himself into my precious things. I was thinking about you, and he picked up the beads and immediately

put them around his neck. He was barely a year old and sat there with blond hair shining and the deepest brown eyes you ever saw, so dark they sometimes look black. Please keep the beads.

2. I dreamed I gave you a stone, hanging it around your neck. I found it, or it found me, several years ago, and I have worn it for some time. It has some healing quality for me, but then again I don't know. It is for you to have and hold as long as you need it, then return when you no longer do.

3. And in meditation this morning I saw you very clearly. I couldn't make sense of it—I'm not sure I need to—so I just report what I saw. You were standing in front of me, and it was quite dark all around. Not a fearful dark, but the dark of a deep indigo night. Your right eye was dark, as if empty, and I couldn't make sense of this because you told me the problem was with your left eye, but I kept looking, and the eye that was dark and not seeing was to my left—i.e., your right. There was a strong "voice" saying, repeatedly, "nineteen." . . . And nineteen threads, quite bright and silvery/golden, were radiating from your head like the spokes of a wheel, outward, but coming to a distinct end, at what in measurable terms was maybe a few meters. The threads were unbound, unconnected, at loose ends, in some way . . . I couldn't understand. Hanging straight out, suspended in the air, all in the same plane about the level of your forehead. Only when I looked at you from above did they appear to radiate out like the spokes of a wheel. And all the time "nineteen, nineteen, nineteen," like a mantra. . . . I do not understand; I do my best to simply report.

There is some help coming; be alert, expect.

In love,
Steve

This day, too, I learned from Peggy Burkhardt, a nurse who is also on the editorial board of the *Alternative Therapies* journal, that I have been placed on a worldwide prayer list of Carmelite communities. I'm beginning to think, "Good God in heaven, what can the outcome of my life be with so much prayer going on?" And not infrequently I thought, "I am not worthy."

I receive a message the next day from Stan Krippner. He is another lifeline. I learned how to teach by watching him; now I learn how to give support in crisis.

> Don't waste your energy answering all these "get-well" messages, but I am still hanging in there for you, praying, lighting candles, sending energy every day. Lots of other people are doing the same, and I am spreading the word.
>
> Love,
> Stan

I write back, and as I read my response, I remember the vacuum I felt:

> Dear Stan:
> Thanks again for being there. I am still in limbo. I am not a good patient, am not sick, can see perfectly well to get around, and am getting bored with being so self-absorbed. The irony is that one of the biggest supporters of alternative therapies has a problem that can only be treated by the highest-tech science in the world and is so rare that there are few statistics and almost no clinical trials. There are only two or three nuclear reactors in the country used for medical purposes, and I need one of them. My penchant for drama, I guess. I will keep you posted. When the actual treatment is decided, I will ask for a "healing web." I am not incapacitated, except by fear.

From Steve Wright, a follow-up to his E-mail of two days ago: "And in the dream last night, you again with nineteen radiating threads and an endlessly repeating: 'There is a jewel in your forehead, turn, turn, like the wheel, turn, turn.' I only pass on what I see or hear. I do not know what it means."

I write back: "I am taking this dream into my dreams. What I got last night was an urgency to connect something, that something had been disconnected. It felt as if either a circle or a necklace had been broken. I just report also."

This is the way ancient medicine works: you share dream space, you dream and redream for one another, and out of the dreams comes "medicine."

———◇———

The mistletoe arrives, seven tiny ampoules in a small white box. One is to be injected every other day. The first dose is the most diluted, and the strength of the mistletoe builds up over time. I'd injected animals thousands of times, but shooting yourself up falls into a slightly different category. Like insulin, the mistletoe is supposed to be shot subcutaneously (under the skin), and diabetics often inject their legs. Trouble is, I don't have much skin or fat on my legs, so the first series is awful. I am probably shooting it into muscle. My legs get swollen, and welts develop around the injection sites. It isn't long before I run out of leg and waddle when I walk.

I used imagery every time I injected mistletoe. I held the syringe and thanked the plant and then thanked Rudolf Steiner, the visionary who started prescribing it maybe fifty years ago, and then I did a little prayer while injecting it. I imagined it moving rapidly through my body, stimulating the immune cells, and heading straight for the Thing and attacking it directly.

———◇———

Near the end of the first week in September, the radionics lady calls. Matters are basically better, the vitality scale is up, the Eye Thing is resolving, but my liver is toxic. I decide to stop her treatments for now and resume them later, just because the cost of everything is adding up. Today I feel flulike. (Elevated temperature and flu symptoms can be expected a few hours after injecting mistletoe.) I am down to one coffee break a day and up a few more enzymes.

A physician colleague calls and sets me back into the fear space. She thinks I should just go to Massachusetts Eye and Ear and get the tumor removed and then proceed with whatever alternatives. She expresses her opinion in no uncertain terms and sounds like my mother. She doesn't listen long enough to hear that it is not a simple matter of having the tumor removed. The eye goes with it. Later she writes me an apology for having been so opinionated without sufficient information.

Her response was not uncommon and was why I didn't tell many people about what I was doing. I would get lectures—well-intentioned, I have no doubt—because I made people nervous with my creative, nonsanctioned regimen. When I made them nervous, they made me crazy, and it often blindsided me (another expression that gets my attention). A woman who is very involved in the alternative and complementary medicine movement, and also familiar with conventional medicine, asked, "I was wondering when you are finally going to decide to get curative treatment." I was exhausted from searching for effective therapies and too frustrated to answer. If there was a cure, I would be first in line.

——◇——

I travel to California, via Dallas, and speak to the Peacemaker Group—all women—at Our Lady of Guadelupe Church on September 8. At the end of my presentation, I get a standing ovation and am moved to tears. My heart is still in the refugee camps, and many of the women in the audience have had similar experiences. The woman-woman connection is electric, an outpouring of love.

Jo Wharton, a friend from Dallas, led me into the small Guadelupe Chapel and gave me roses. (One remained on my altar at home for more than a year.) Don Campbell left me a message at the hotel: "May the great Goddesses of Light and the God of Corn from his haughty Palaces chiming forth with choirs of tambourines be with you."

As I walked from the church back to the Fairmont Hotel carrying the roses, it began to rain. A collective shout went up in Dallas. It was the first rain in sixty-five days. I was thinking about the strange dream I was living in: back in Dallas, my old stomping ground, it was raining, and I was carrying roses from the Guadelupe Church to the Fairmont Hotel—and who *is* writing this story?

Mistletoe number 3, the third vial, on the fifth day since beginning the injections. Now I know I'm hitting muscle. Big red welts. My energy is pretty damn good, but I am tired of all this. (Boy, in retrospect, it was pretty early to start getting tired.)

Off to California and adventures of a serious spiritual nature.

Shamanic Healing

{September 8}

MO AND MARA JAN were my partners on this journey to the world of shamanism. We left from Mo's on the afternoon of September 8, drove to Sonoma, and checked into a spa. Figured we might as well get some body work and other spalike things done during the day, before we did the spiritual healing thing at night.

The time is auspicious. Most of the New Agers think the world is coming to an end tomorrow—on 9/9/99. A physicist from Germany went to the Peacemakers conference in Dallas because it was for women, and the eighth of September was to be the most powerful day of feminine energy in history—or so he said. I tried to understand what he based his thinking on, but it seemed to be some revealed information. Hot days to trot, anyhow, for metaphysics.

We drove up to Michael and Sandy Harner's home at dusk. The air was charged and smelled like ozone. There were flashes of lightning. You only have to have lived in California for a short while to know that there are rarely lightning displays like those great Midwest and Texas storms, and there is never rain in September. Not the season. It rains in the late winter and spring. It was so unexpected and out of place that we almost didn't notice it. What's the old story about Cortés or Vasco da Gama or one of the explorers? The natives saw his ship, but they didn't really *see* it because they'd never seen a ship before. Something goofy happens in the brain when we try to process truly unrecognizable material. That's what happened with the storm. It didn't compute.

The weather drama made headlines: SURPRISE THUNDERSTORM ROLLS THROUGH BAY AREA. From the *San Francisco Chronicle:* "Hundreds of lightning bolts lit the night sky as heavy downpours continued on and off for hours in some areas." A meteorologist was quoted as saying it was the "most spectacular electrical storm we've had in at least two decades." A sheriff's dispatcher described bolts that touched ground: "They came in back to back to back: boom, boom, boom."

I clipped several articles from the paper the next day. Thirty thousand people were without power. The storm went on most of the night, crackling, popping, and pumping out smells. I'll just say one more thing about it before we get to the healing work. Shamans are known for using, shall we say, "special effects" to stimulate the power of belief. They are also reputed to be able to cause weather changes. When we were in the house, I actually thought it might be possible that Michael was using some light display tactics. The lightning just never stopped. Was it lightning? Lightning doesn't act like that. The room—lit only by a single candle—was flooded with light.

I simply don't remember everything about these three nights. Shamanism has been a spiritual practice for me for a long while, so the ceremonies themselves were no surprise. Michael's pure, pristine access to the spirit world was. He lifted a veil, and immediately we all stepped into the place of spirit. The total sense of love in the room was also a surprise: every act, every word was filled with unconditional love. We all loved one another, of course—we are mostly old friends—but this energy was bigger than friendship.

Sandy Harner, Mo, Mara Jan, and I sit in the living room while Michael takes a little time alone. Their home is modern, aesthetically pleasing, and very uncluttered. There is a notable absence of shamanic props or bric-a-brac. Michael comes in, as he does for the next nights, and lights a candle and a fat stick of woody incense. Sandy and Mo drum for a short while at his suggestion. He invites the spirits to join us. They do. I don't see these things (maybe after my initiation into the Underworld I will) but could feel them and knew what they were. I feel polar bear and skunk and later ask who invited them. It was Mara Jan. She always does, she says. Spirits surround us. Michael talks to me for a few minutes, and I go over the diagnosis, my strange summer, and the "soul loss" from so many things, but especially my children. Michael is quiet, listening to someone or something we cannot hear, and then says, "The spirits say you have more of their work to do here." That's not bad for starters. Sounds as if I'm going to be around a few more years, and life is getting slightly more interesting than it was before the Eye Thing.

Michael places a small rug in the middle of the floor and asks me to lie down. I think he lies beside me, and there is more drumming. He then sits behind me and cups my eye—the "good" eye—with his hand. He does some extractions from my face and head. (Extractions involve sucking or pulling out entities that are causing disease and are a common shamanic practice.) He also does some water purification, asking me to drink a glass of spring water and throwing some in my face. It startles me and gets in my eyes. While I am on the floor, though, it feels as if the winds come through the house. Lightning and now wind. The candle flame dances. There is wind, by God, I'm not making this up. It stops when I sit up and go back to the sofa.

Michael then brings out two stools. They look ancient, like something that shamans in Siberia or someplace had sat on at the beginning of time. We sit facing each other. He asks me to put "Jeanne" aside and, if there is anyone else inhabiting my body, to let that person speak. I am too self-conscious to do this well and refuse to make anything up. What comes to me, though, is a young woman, thirty-six years old, called "Mamacita." She is standing in a doorway to a simple house and looking out across a barren piece of land. I can get no further. Michael does more "traveling" himself, and the spirits give him a healing song for me: "Halo through [pause] light." He does not know what it could mean, and neither do I, except that it is significant. Off and on since, I have used it as a mantra. These are the main things I remember from the first night. Michael then asks the spirits to stay in the room until we come back.

The second night I made a very conscious decision to stay out of the way as much as possible, meaning that I wasn't going to pull my usual control-freak number and try to make something happen. I needed to release all expectations, all need for control, and stay open to the experience. We repeat several of the ceremonies of the previous night. I talk about the darkness in my life, how haunted I feel in my home, the large number of Black Madonnas that have been given to me and surround me, my experience at the feet of the Black Madonna of Poland.

I do not tell Michael all of the story, only the outline, but for the record, here is what happened, because it is rather interesting, at least to me. Quite by "accident" (ha-ha), Mo, Judy, Carl Simonton, Marius Wirga, and I were in Częstochowa, Poland, the night when the Black Madonna's feast day was being celebrated and the service broadcast throughout the world. We were on our way to teach in southern Poland and had stopped there for the night. We happened to go into the church in the late afternoon and sat in the small alcove where the icon is hung. Except for special occasions, she is veiled. Tons of amber beads are strung across the altar, and there are gifts from the pope himself. The screen lifted, and we saw the most famous Black Madonna in the world, holding her child, and dressed in gilt and jewels for the occasion. When we turned to leave, we saw thousands of people crowding the main church, the grounds, and lined up and down the streets, and we, of course, not wanting to miss a party and being unable to get out anyway, stayed.

This Black Madonna is credited with having saved the country from Huns, Swedes, and numerous other invading hordes and has been carried into battle for hundreds of years. The Huns desecrated her by slashing her face to steal power from her and the country. She is the Madonna of sorrow, regardless of whatever else she might be. I affectionately called her the "kick-butt" Madonna, because she means business. She is not the smiling, gentle Mary the Mother of Jesus. The Mother of the Earth, some say she is, but I don't know.

Mo nearly had apoplexy (if that is still a diagnosis) as churchmen in fancy gold and blue lamé gowns gathered about the altar, while quite a few of them spoke. The churchwomen, who were not allowed in this consecrated space, instead crawled on their hands and knees around the altar and behind it to pay homage to one of their own. But I digress.

So, in putting this into some perspective about women and children, I also tell Michael that part of our property in New Mexico is a burial ground and no buildings will ever be allowed between the neighbors and us. The die is therefore cast: I've been surrounding myself with the collective sorrow of mothers and their children, with a few other issues about women and their men thrown in for good measure.

As Michael works on this second night, we all hear rain, and Sandy rushes around to close the windows. But there is no rain. The wind blows across me as I lie on the floor. Michael instructs Mara Jan to move—she seems to be blocking something. Actually she is between the ocean and us, and it could have been that the negative entities were being cast oceanward, which would not be unusual.

Michael talks about the cross-cultural use of icons. He says they were often used to take away pain and suffering and were damaged deliberately in the area where a healing was being requested. He thinks that Christ is such an icon but the message got confused over time. He suggests I might look for an icon suitable for healing my eye.

The spirits are asked to remain until the next night, and we girls drive back to Sonoma, where another miracle occurs: we are prepared a delicious meal even though the kitchen is officially closed. We obviously looked starved and the chef took pity.

The final night Michael has invited in a very well-known and highly skilled medium, whom I'll call Jack. We begin the ceremony as we have on previous nights, speaking our intentions, acknowledging the spirits. The veil has parted; we are There again. The telephone rings, and the voice on the answering machine is Frank's, wondering where I was because the hotel/spa had no record of my having checked in two days ago.

Jack stays in the kitchen for about an hour and is then invited into the room with the rest of us. The air in the room is dense, thick, highly energized, as one might expect with so many spirits around. We have become slightly acclimated, but Jack has not. He seems to become faint or ill as he enters the room, and Sandy brings him some water. Jack breathes rapidly and finally settles into the chair. With Jack facing away from me, Michael asks me again to step aside and allow any others who may be harboring themselves within my body to come forth. One comes immediately—Lucita. She seems to be from some time past, lives near the water, but says, "There is another one here, too." It is the "other one" whom I am instructed not to encourage back.

She will not speak to Michael but finally addresses Sandy. The voice coming from Jack is that of a woman. My body does something it has never done before: it shivers and moves, and I cannot stop it. Whatever is happening is visceral. Something very dark seems to pass through me and then out. The message from whatever the hell this was is that my kindness has made me an open vessel for the suffering souls of the world—dead or alive. I am kind, the desire to be kind drives my life and intentions, and this must be given some thought.

Michael has obviously given the medium information before we got there. Jack volunteers his belief that I need to get the icons out of the house as soon as possible. "And the burial ground?" I ask. They agree that I should honor the dead, take flowers, and make a little ceremony as often as I can but that the house itself did not have to be a problem forever. We could live there, cleanse, and honor the beautiful land. I had not done that.

"And what about Lucita?" This is the beginning of many references to a Lucinda, a Lucy, the patron of vision. She seemed to be with me in a healing fashion. Life is strange. I had only recently remembered that Saint Lucy was chosen for the cover of my book *Woman as Healer,* Lucy with the shamanic feather and holding a pair of eyes.

Michael decides to do a little soul retrieval—a journey to the shamanic world to bring back a piece of me that has taken flight. Sometimes this comes in the form of an animal, as when Sandy Ingerman did her work a few weeks before and found the eagle for me. Usually the animal represents a part of you that has been stolen, lost, or just abandoned. Like a piece that is young, courageous, hopeful, or in my case just plain fun. Life goes on, and these things get lost. Mo and Sandy drum but, as usual, not for long. Michael returns from his trance journey and says he found a beaver. Jesus H. God. A beaver. I wonder whether it could be a power animal of some kind, but he shakes his head, no, he'd never actually found a beaver during a soul retrieval before.

Mo and I shriek and nearly wet our pants. "Lightning Beaver" had been my secret name because of certain earlier propensities to enjoy physical encounters often and with some remarkable speed. Entirely unwomanly, I suppose, but that is the way it was, and I usually did not apologize until recently. Well, anyhow, they all drum, and I dance the Beaver—a happy, social, energetic, life-celebrating dance that makes Mo cry. Beaver needs to come back to life.

As we leave the final session and are making our good-byes, Michael says, "But there is something I don't get. It seemed like the beaver

came from a medieval period. There were bridges and construction."
Of course.

I tell him about the last time I saw the Beaver, an unforgettable time
in Munich, Germany, a few years ago. Mo, Frank, Carl, and I were
joined by Mo's wild Austrian lover, Richard, who looks like a handsome
pirate, is about seven feet tall, and knows every single great wine and
restaurant in Europe. We'd been working in Europe for about a month
and needed a little holiday. We had good intentions as we strolled out
of the Four Seasons Hotel: we tried to tour some churches, but they
were all closed for repairs, and the museums were either closed or too
far away.

It was Christmas market time, so the inner city was a giant fair. Richard stopped frequently to purchase rounds of mead, the old Viking
drink, which we just had to pour into the bushes occasionally when his
back was turned. Mead, fermented from honey, will make you nuts. We
got enough down, though, to make it one of the most festive days in
our history. A Russian violinist played sad love songs on the street corner, and I have a picture of the five of us moved to tears under three
black umbrellas. Frank, who had just taken a quick trip to Japan and
back, passed out every time we sat down, face in his plate of bratwurst,
of which we ate quite a few.

During this holiday we shared secret names, and my totem—the
truth of the joyful, spontaneous part of me—was revealed to one and
all. I was Lightning Beaver. Since my lifetime sexual partners can be
counted on the fingers of one hand (and two of those were so bad I'm
leaving them out), it was a well-guarded secret. After a suitable period of stunned silence, there was an uproar of backslapping and foot
stomping.

As we left the restaurant, we saw a glass case, there in the middle of
downtown Munich, right in front of us, containing a stuffed beaver.
What are the odds? Beavers don't even live in Europe anymore. I took
a picture, lest this seem too unbelievable.

Beavers were sent my way after this—a crystal one from Austria, two
purple ones carved from precious stones. They are in my treasure chest,
long forgotten because Beaver has not made many appearances the past
few years.

"Of course, Michael, the last time that beaver showed up, we were in Munich, Germany. It did look medieval, and the downtown was full of construction."

Three days of shamanic healing, starting with Lightning and ending with Beaver. Pretty darn amazing.

Girl Talk

{September 10}

WE TRAVELED BACK to Mo's for the night and got there around midnight. Mara Jan felt compelled to tell me something. Years ago, she said, she idolized me. I had everything, was the epitome of what she wanted to be (which at this writing I am not certain was what).

She was helping Mo with her research for her dissertation (which I chaired) on the brain effects of listening to drumming, especially the type used in shamanic work. I had volunteered to be one of the test subjects. The study involved measuring electronic brain waves using an electroencephalograph (EEG), and it took hours to put electrodes on the scalps of the subjects. Some guy who owned the equipment insisted on a presession that lasted forever (against my better judgment), and you stayed wired up for hours. I was completely oblivious to Mara Jan, who was putting on and taking off the electrodes. Furthermore, I jerked the electrodes off midway through the study and left. My doggy, Sasha, was at home dying from complications of diabetes. All I could think about was getting home to her. She had cried all night, and I couldn't bear to hear her in such pain. We had her put gently to sleep the next day.

I really didn't see Mara Jan, and I really didn't mean to be rude. To get back at me for being such a disappointment, she decided to go flirt with Frank. She said she wasn't especially attracted to him, didn't know him at all, and was just interested in retaliation. Well, holy shit. How often had this happened?

I am very glad Mara Jan told me; it was a major healing for her and a new awareness for me. There were always flirtations going on around Frank, and of course, I first blamed him and the women, and later I blamed myself for being so inadequate that the doorway of seduction always appeared open. Mara Jan's confession shed a new light on this vile old pattern, and my female nature received a little balm.

On my way home the following day, I write in my poorly kept journal, "God's blessings are great—I have work to do—let me be worthy. I need quiet time and guidance, a 'Seeing Eye dog.' " Some visionary powers seem to have been granted, and just in time. I note that something different and active—lightninglike—has been happening in my eye. It is a little disorienting.

I make a note that there is no garbage in Michael's work; he effortlessly goes straight to spirit. My intellect has become boring, and feeling abused is getting oppressive and not dignified. Fuck it. Time for a new vision. My mantra is, "When my Vision returns, my vision will return. Halo through. Light." I also write, "Let's allow this life to unfold a little more; without fear it can be done. Not so much hiding and sleeping." I mention Frank: "When I am really fearful, I need to be held by him, and this may not be fair. He may be too overwhelmed and fragile himself. Is it fair to ask him to be a companion on this healing journey? I don't know. My greatest fear was that he would die and I would have to live alone. Now I am afraid he will have to care for me, and it won't work. He can't. I can't. I don't think we can change this without serious intentions."

Detective Work

{September 12}

HOME TODAY. I decided to pick some flowers and place them in the arroyo and the burial site. I asked the spirits (or whomever) to give me a sign that my efforts were not silly and wasted. As I looked down, I saw a cervical vertebra on a flat rock. It was human and from a small child, the first bone I'd ever found on this property. I gave it to Mo. The Saturday before I got home, Frank had found a skunk skin in the hobby shop. For no good reason, he decided to buy it. It went to Mara Jan. My thank-you to both of them for their presence on this unbelievable journey.

From the next day on, until I left for England on September 19, events were trying. I realized I had very little but my intuition to go on, and I knew I'd weasel out of or delay the medical treatment that was being offered in any way I could.

I have had a recurrent dream for as long as I can remember. I am in a hospital at night, and surgery is planned for the next day. I rethink the whole business and can't imagine why I'd agreed to it in the first place. I leave the hospital in the middle of the night.

Today I throw the *I Ching*. I ask what my stance should be toward medical treatment and throw number 5—Waiting! I ask what my treatment should be and throw number 39—Obstruction. Obstacles surround me, but these can be overcome. Pause in view of danger and then retreat. I must join forces with friends of like mind and put myself under the leadership of people equal to the purpose. This requires the will to persevere just when one apparently must do something that leads away from the goal. This time is useful for self-development. This is the value of adversity.

———◇———

Continuing with my medical inquiry, I call Andy Weil. He recommends mushrooms, and I order them posthaste, to arrive before I leave for England. He also suggests some Chinese healers, but quite honestly, I'm feeling the need to put a stop to the nonstop remedies. I don't trust all the materials being imported from China right now, anyway, because many contain pesticides and heavy metals. More pills from Ed Tyska arrive.

The mistletoe skin reaction is huge. I have the flu. The injection sites look like bee stings. I do two shamanic journeys during the day. The message from the journeys is "Go in peace; be prepared." I do the kill-or-cure routine—injections, coffee breaks, sauna, and the several thousand supplements (I exaggerate, but not by much)—for the rest of the week. I feel heat on the left side of my face. This will be my only sign of immune activity for two months.

———◇———

I get a psychic reading from a well-known so-called medical intuitive. The message: The eye knows how to heal itself. Cancer feeds on fear and doubt. Get rid of old trash in my life. I know she is highly regarded, but I'm not sure how much was my stuff and how much hers. She says there was a turning point when I was eight and I need to revisit that time. She says my father had a tremendous dislike for me and knew I saw right through him. He is saying, "I know better now." I should praise Frank more, she says; my fame has been hard on him, and he believes he would have been more famous had it not been for me. But he loves me deeply. He doesn't know how to help me right now.

My daughter doesn't like me much because she's jealous, I'm a rival, and she is reaching out for help. My son is troubled but being cleansed now. She says my eyes have seen too much and I should not have gone to Macedonia: the work with the Kosovars interfered with some karmic script. The eye speaks with a penetrating gaze, and I looked too deeply into problems but did not take precautions to protect myself from projections. I am being tested to believe in myself and, in doing so, am stripping myself. I need to talk to my eye, abstain from challenges. The heart will tell the truth. I need to meditate on my heart, and I will know when the treatment is correct. Put my hand over my heart, she said. Trust. Buy time before treatment. She said my head was a library full of information and I needed to let some of it go. I was not going to die from this.

I did not find the reading especially helpful at the time, but later it did initiate the decision to explore those mysteriously difficult years of my childhood.

On this fifteenth day of September, I call Massachusetts Eye and Ear to schedule something, anything—an evaluation, a treatment. The very nice person on the other end of the line goes through the treatment protocol. Obviously they have a plan and are not completely at the mercy of the defense needs of the nuclear reactor. Rhonda Fleck, the oncologist and friend here in Santa Fe, has already called about the radiation oncologist and learned he is a nice man. Nice is good. The West Coast girlfriends say they can go East, if need be, and I should get the best treatment, wherever it may be. The man who is in charge of the big treatment is out for three weeks.

"Yippee," I write. "The angel is taking care of me. Otherwise, I might feel compelled to hop a plane and get my eye smoked out instead of going to England. I'm happy." I have a good, long nap and a productive shamanic journey. Frank and I have dinner and a good talk. I have the feeling today that this nasty Thing will go away. I have time. Zillions of prayers are headed heavenward for me.

About this time I made other calls, one of them to B. R. Ksander at Harvard. He is one of a rare breed of specialists on immunology of the eye. I have also found some of his articles on the Web, where he and his colleagues discuss their findings that ocular melanomas accumulate lymphocytes (white blood cells) with the potential to kill tumor cells. Their results imply that if the cytotoxic cells (cellular killers) could be activated within the progressively growing ocular tumors, it might be possible to eliminate the tumor cells.

August (Al) Reader, a neuroophthalmologist in San Francisco, paves the way by calling Ksander first and telling him of my situation and my interests. Al is one of my ocular lifelines: he has written about the sacred nature of the eye, his own near-death experiences, and the visual pathways of meditation. He, like so many, made himself available to me whenever and for whatever. He has encouraged most of what I have done, sent me articles on spontaneous remissions of ocular melanomas, and reframed some of my symptoms for me that could represent healing, but I know that he, too, must be uncomfortable about the fact that I eventually exited the traditional system. Maybe I shouldn't second-guess him, though.

I ask Ksander a few blunt questions about why there have been no attempts to put his findings into clinical practice. He explains to me the difference between clinical and experimental medicine! I don't need this explanation—I know you can't just jump findings from the mouse lab into the hospital—but it is curious that more tentative clinical trials, specific to ocular melanoma, have not begun.

What he tells me is that there are tumor-infiltrating lymphocytes harvested from somebody's tumor that have the capacity to kill tumor cells in other people, and I guess these are probably stashed in a refrigerator somewhere. When I tell him the names of the doctors with whom I have consulted, he says, "Remember that each one of these doctors has only one or two tools and will try to sell you on them."

Rain Borden, a nurse everyone hopes to have by their side if they perchance wind up in the cardiovascular intensive care unit, sends me an article about Ram Dass. He calls his stroke "tough grace." He is my hero. I quoted him to him at a dinner party a few years back, and when we were housed in rooms next to each other in a retreat, I thought life just couldn't get any better.

Today I try to remember last spring. I can't. This makes me crazy. Sometimes I try to remember every minute of my life. Figure it is good exercise for the mind. I get out the calendar to see when I went to Monterey. I can't figure it all out. I have a garden, so I must have gone to stores, planted, fertilized, watered. I must also have brought in truckloads of soil, or I wouldn't be doing anything but trying to grow plants on beds of rock. Flowers and weeds and vegetables have come up. The flowers are feral. I like that word *feral*. Maybe I'm feral, too, so there is no coincidence here; all us feral folks just hang in there.

———◇———

Slept and meditated all day on September 16 and didn't answer the telephone. My fever went way up, and I shot mistletoe in the afternoon. I do have the self-induced flu—as good an excuse as any to stay in bed. The medical intuitive said to rest the eye and let it take care of itself. I will try to rest, but tomorrow is busy. Life gets better, strangely. I see more beauty and excitement. Am truly excited about England.

———◇———

I write what I need: a compound to live in, an assistant to help me with the many details of my life, a release of the need to keep up with science (I just can't do it all), a puppy, a book to write, and Frank—the brilliant, loving man I married—returned to me.

———◇———

Margaret Christensen comes to my home bearing gifts. She has made me an exquisite lacquered box with Saint Lucy on the cover and animals decoupaged around the sides. Sand from the healing church at Chimayó is sprinkled into the varnish. Inside the lid a is a round mirror, and in the box are seeds from wildflowers. It becomes my portable shrine, heavy though it is; I refuse ever to check it with luggage. Margaret also has a story: She was in the Guadelupe Chapel in Dallas the week before and noticed a vintage picture of Saint Lucy. The caretaker of the chapel is a patient of hers, so she asked her what happened to the votives and gifts left at the altar. "Oh, we just give them away finally when someone seems to need them." The Saint Lucy picture had been "dropped off" by a woman who was moving. "Give it to someone who needs her." So there I have her—another Saint Lucy—in the bedroom about to become a shrine room.

England: A Healing Pilgrimage

{September 19}

I HAVE BEEN UP most of the night, wired, and am feeling lousy as Frank takes me to the airport. Trying to tie up the loose ends of my jobs, pack, and get the gear organized for several workshops takes days of concentration, and I'm never sure I'll be able to get the suitcases closed before the plane leaves. Why don't I just stay home and be sick? Boring, that's why. Mo and Judy pick me up at San Jose. I've really made a mess of things this time. I sit down on the floor in Mo's kitchen and try to repack, and with everything out on the floor, it looks as if a bag lady were going through the trash. It's obvious I need another suitcase, which Mo lends me. I just can't seem to get everything done right anymore.

Bob Bischoff, craftsman par excellence, has just produced his finest piece of art: an icon of Saint Lucy for me to take on my pilgrimage. She is a beauty—a piece of gently curving wood, holding an eye and a candle. She is my most prized possession. I know I am supposed to deface her eye, but on such a work of art, it feels like sacrilege. I poke at it a little, then wrap her carefully to be my constant companion, and she travels like a doll in the shrine box from Margaret.

———◇———

Each day now is a step along a healing pilgrimage. Time outside of time. It has holy moments and sometimes entire hours of holiness. Judy is the best of the best traveling companions. Being with her is an astonishing experience, and I can hardly wait until mornings so we can catch up on dreams, moan, cackle, slug down the coffee, and do the "organ recital" as Ram Dass calls it, going over our pains from the night before. She's a joyful, selfless, kindred soul. She's also naughty, and so am I—or I used to be. Judy's blue eyes are clear and bright anytime, even after long hours on an airplane, and she usually has a little collection of men around her. Even the man who gonged the dinner bell at a castle we stayed at hit on her when we found him, drunk as a skunk, in the back hallway.

On the way to London, Judy and I settled ourselves into our exceptionally comfortable business-class seats. We had a little champagne, followed by some reasonable, slightly gourmet food, but nothing that could account for how terrible we felt when we got to London. I can truly say I have never felt so bad in my life up until then, but as you may have guessed, it did get worse. I felt as if I were on fire, but it was *cold* fire. I'm a physiologist, remember, but nothing in the annals of medicine or biology accounted for this abysmal condition. Maybe it was the damn mushrooms. I had bolted down quite a few on the plane. These were organically grown but certainly not clinically evaluated or tested in any way to my knowledge. Keep in mind that this is self-experimentation. Maybe it is not such a hot idea to take mushrooms and mistletoe, both poisons, at the same time or on an airplane? Or maybe, and quite likely, all that mistletoe I'd been shooting into my leg muscles had just started to circulate. Became convinced only an emergency liver transplant would save me. Fortunately I went to sleep.

We finally get to the hotel and pass out in a temporary room. It is only seven in the morning, and our real rooms are not available. Judy runs me a bath—my first clue that I am going to learn to allow myself to be cared for on this trip. The hotel has no record of my reservations. This is the second time this month: Sonoma Inn, where we stayed for the Harner shamanic adventure, didn't either. Maybe I've already departed to the Great Beyond and the girlfriends are just humoring me. We make a feeble attempt to walk on Bond Street, eat lunch, and then I simply must crawl into bed. Judy feels awful, too, but being the sport she is, she takes to the street. In a store she meets an American who tells her to go to bed. "You always have to go to bed in the afternoon when you take that flight. Take a four-hour nap, eat dinner, and go back to bed." Judy returns and flops next to me.

———◇———

On September 21 we do London. Doing London for eight hours when you're sick as a horse is quite an event. My energy is fine, my feet and legs hold out, I'm just on cold fire, and aspirin helps. Later I learned that "cold fire" was probably the immune system going full throttle. The chemicals of immunity are toxic, they kill cells, and they feel as if they're killing you—trust me on this one. I've never felt anything like it before. It is not a fever as we know it. For God's sake, we need to start recording this, describing the phenomena, as they say. This was a small preview of what would send me into shock two months later.

We walk forever. I've ratcheted up my pain threshold (ratcheting up is becoming a specialty) out of sheer, stubborn determination to experience the pleasure of the day. Then we go to see where Ann Boleyn was beheaded. She was a Butler, and I fancy her distantly related on my mother's side of the family and am secretly proud to be of her lineage. A woman who spoke her mind. Well, maybe once or twice too often.

Judy and I have a great talk about kindness and how we may have learned it as a result of early abuse—either a defense or an exceptional sensitivity. Judy is the kindest person I know.

We had planned to go to the theater that night. I neglected to tell her I hate the theater. I sleep during the theater. I'm thinking, for Judy I'm gonna give it a try. At dinner I tell her the awful truth: I can't make it. She chastises me for my lack of honesty. Righto. Bad move. I tried to please and then backed down. Then she invites the very cute concierge to go with her! He gracefully declines. I try to write, doze, and decide to shoot mistletoe abdominally. Surprise. It doesn't hurt. Maybe I'm onto something. I pray for progress in vision in three days. It doesn't happen. My entry ends with the mantra "Halo through. Light."

———◇———

Two days later we take the rail to Glastonbury. Between us we have close to two thousand pounds of luggage, and train travel is going to be quite the effort. Luckily we are both strong, and the British males—even the old coots—are helpful. What I didn't know at the time was that Judy was carrying heavy bottles of sweet pickles, for crying out loud. Our sponsor, hostess, and girlfriend, Jean Sayre-Adams, had told her that one of the items she had sorely missed since moving to England was sweet pickles.

Being in Glastonbury is like strolling through a deck of tarot cards. Everyone is in costume. It is a sacred site for religions so old they have no name. Sacred sites always attract "cultural creatives," and the magnetism of this site seems to have intensified over the last ten years. It is full of crystal shops and (I guess) trust-fund babies with dreadlocks and babies of their own. We stay at #3 (yes, that is the name) on the grounds of the old abbey where Arthur and Guinevere are supposed to be buried—and even if they're not, it still has plenty of history. I can see the ruins at night from my bedroom. It is the autumnal full moon, and you could have read a book outside.

The waters from the Chalice Well have an especially long healing history. They contain iron, so the rocks are stained red. Blood of the Mother, for sure. We visit the well twice, touched to tears each time, and collect bottles of water to give to our friends. I have about half a bottle left. It is part of my anointing solution, and come spring, I will pour it into my fishpond.

It is a wonder how anyone can keep up with Judy's energy, but mostly I managed. Bet we walked thirty miles a day. We walked up to the Tor, the remains of an ancient tower atop a hill that is Glastonbury's major landmark, as the sun was setting. It was a steep, windy, and very cold climb, which gave us a glimpse of the mists of Avalon and where the book by that name was conceived.

The first morning we walk out of #3, we cross the street to the old poorhouse. Now this is a really *old* poorhouse. Probably tenth-century. It had housed about eleven men, whose care was paid for by the not-insignificant funds from the abbey. It is now a chapel and a museum. A man walks out. "Hello. I'm Brian. I'm a Druid." We have our pictures taken with Brian and his walking stick and his healing stick. Two sticks, both decked out in gemstones. Whether Brian is a Druid or what a Druid might be in this day and age is beside the point. He has a great outfit. Judy takes my picture in a decrepit chapel, where I'm sitting on the floor beside a hand-lettered sign: THE PEOPLE WALKING IN DARK-NESS HAVE SEEN A GREAT LIGHT. I forgot at the time that it is from the Bible ("The people who walk in darkness will see a great light—a light that will shine on all who live in the land where death casts its shadow"—Isaiah 9:2, New Living Translation) and that I had sung those words for so many years in choirs.

At this point I certainly had no idea what that great light might be, but I knew I was in darkness, in the land where death cast its shadow, and was moving toward something.

A couple of more mistletoe injections and that's it for the series, for now. I've given up on the kill-or-cure routine in the interests of time and space and mostly am only taking enzymes. I try to talk Judy into sampling the mushrooms to see whether they would affect her. She hauls along a suitcase full of supplements when she travels—but nope, not the mushrooms. Some experiments you can't even count on your best friends for.

The little period starts again and makes me very distracted and nervous. I'm dying, I just know it. I'm either going to have a stroke, bleed to death, have my organs malfunction, or just plain scare the wits out of myself. Because my depth perception is gradually getting more and more fucked, touring the sites is also making me nervous. Death would be easier, I'm thinking again. But not until after this pilgrimage.

What I am noticing is that I'm curious again. When the curiosity died, I started dimming, or maybe it was the other way around. And I'm starting to laugh. Most of the things, you had to be there to see the humor (as with Brian), but I'm chuckling now and then, and the sound seems a little foreign.

———◇———

The area around #3 and the abbey grounds is notorious for being a place of dreams and visions. Whatever dream maker abides on that land must have facilitated dreams that repeated themselves in some form for the next year and became so persistent that they permeated my waking consciousness. I dreamed I was in a house and found my birds. In this dream they were in an attic, and J.C. was carrying a rag doll like a baby. The number of birds had actually multiplied, and although they were not in great health, they were alive. Frank had known about their being there all along and had been sporadically feeding and cleaning them.

Then I had a second dream, in which I was asleep and heard voices in the driveway. Frank had brought home many houseguests. I had not invited them, nor did I recognize their faces. I tried to find beds for them and was surprised and relieved to discover that I had so much room.

So after that I often dreamed about the birds and about coming home to houseguests or a house packed with people I did not recognize. Sometimes I am fairly lucid or half awake during the latter dream and am amazed at how I could look at so many people, with their features so clear, and not recognize a single one of them. Occasionally I will ask them who they are and what they are doing in my house. Each has a different reason. I ask myself how a mind can do this in dreams because, awake, I could not conjure up these faces. The home-invasion dreams feel more like time warps than dreams—as if I'd entered into another time and witnessed actual events.

———◇———

The enchanted dream maker on this holy land is still working, and I feel more compelled to record dreams than the daily activities. I had another house dream the following night. We were landscaping, and I was finding all sorts of plants, an ivy tripod, and paths. Lush, as in English gardens. Frank and I were transferring the fish while we cleaned the pond. They had gotten very large. We put them in a bag, and they died. The beautiful white one lived longer, but its gills were also chewed up. I was sorry but said we could find more fish. I don't quite know what to think of this dream.

We actually did buy a white coy last summer after I had a dream that a big white fish was unraveling the DNA on the Thing. We called him "Mac," for macrophage. The fish all died a year later, strangely, quickly, and my last image of them was the white coy, slowly swimming in circles. I turned away, unable to bear watching another pet die.

In the garden (in the dream) we were looking at straw bales that supported a garage and found huge quantities of marijuana stalks. They were moldy and of no use for recreational purposes. I tried to pull them out but realized the bales were vital to the structure. One could analyze the daylights out of this one: useless dead debris that held the long-lost potential for pleasure and visions, now holding up a structure nevertheless.

I had an awful dream about Chase. It was so bad I didn't tell Judy about it during our dream-processing time at breakfast. He was quite young and was brought home blue. The funeral director came and asked to make arrangements. I was very angry because Chase was not yet dead. I held him astride my hips, and Mel and Frank and I took him to the hospital. I decided that life was not working for him and he needed a different school. He seemed to stay alive.

Another dream. Josefina (my housekeeper) and her mother were cleaning my kitchen. Josefina had just had a new baby girl (and she did, for real). In the dream I offered her all my old baby food in the cupboard, and she started crying, as did her mother. I asked whether the baby was OK, and she said, "Baby OK," but she was adamant that she did not want the food. The sorrow seemed aimed at me, not herself; her tears were not from self-pity but out of some tenderness and compassion she felt for me. I actually did have baby food in the house, jars of peach puree, which I had mixed with the birds' cereal when they were with me. So maybe this, too, was a bird dream. I don't know.

Even with all the dream activity, I had a good night. My vision was weird the previous day, and so was I. It was a mistletoe day, but that didn't seem to account for it. We went to Bath and Wells. I cried at Evensong, especially during the prayers. I realize how intensely I feel sorrow and how little I feel joy, excitement, peace. This is a recurrent theme, and although I can't get rid of it, I'm getting better.

I'm spotting again. Out, out damned spot. On September 24 my vision is a little better—fewer bothersome flashings—although the left side of my face had been numb and tingling only the day before. My body is trying so hard to do something.

Was a great day at the Chalice Well. I felt optimistic, high, and grateful. I am 50 percent convinced this is not "melanoma" but something vascular. I have to stand my ground with the doctors. Explain over and over again, as in my dream last summer, that it is something disconnected.

I write my mantra: "Halo through. Light. Halo through. Light." Whatever it means. . . .

Ceilidh

{September 25}

NOW IT IS TIME to pack up the tonnage and go to Steve Wright's fiftieth birthday celebration, which is held near his home in the Lake District, near Scotland. Again, you had to be there to appreciate all this, and you really had to be an American, because only we know how much trains confuse us. We were on the wrong train, it got to our destination earlier than the planned train, I fell on my butt trying to run out, and Judy couldn't get the door open because we didn't know you have to let the window down and open it from the outside. We did know that the train only stops for a second or two if the door is not opened, and even when it is, you have to jump, so we were a little anxious. It did finally open, and she flew out with it, barely escaping death from disembarkation. Some old gentlemen dressed in wooly things helped us up and out, and handed us our luggage through the rapidly closing door.

We're met by Ian, a friend of Steve's, and whisked away to an old stable decorated for the fiftieth festivities. Food, people, gifts, and a night of the ceilidh, the traditional circle dances. People of all ages from the village dance the old vigorous sets, to the tune of an Irish drum (boron) and a fiddle. A caller announces the dances and calls out the steps, and we weave, move, join arms, do-si-do, bow, hop, form patterns, and let them dissolve and form them again. Quite aerobic, it is, and we end up with at least forty-seven blisters on each foot. Judy and I dance together (you need a partner) and trade off being the guy, but we keep forgetting which of us is supposed to be the guy.

I have house/hotel and kid dreams. Lee Ann is visiting; she leaves fourteen cans of beer in the house and a stack of dirty plates in our hotel room. I try to call her on a funky phone and can't dial the number correctly, which is another frequent dream. (It wouldn't take a wizard to interpret these dreams as a sign that I am frustrated in communicating with my children.) Another dream fragment: Frank and I are taking showers, but separately. The basins are very dirty, full of brown mud that has streamed off of us.

———◇———

Despite the Eye Thing, I feel like myself on the inside. Jeannie's seventeenth-century house has a cozy kitchen conducive to late-night conversations, and we went to bed at one-thirty. Even so, I got up early, drank coffee in bed, and wrote in my journal. I had the best ideas I've had for some time. I am trying to sort things out in my world. The dream material gave some clues. I became conscious of my paralysis for the past two months—just trying to defend myself, to take in information without being taken in. I wrote in my journal: "How can I consciously plan a rich life to live into? Why do I deaden myself, sleep, hide from Frank? Does he want me gone? How would I ever know if he never says anything, which he doesn't?

"No mistletoe today. Will do whatever I can not to feel bad. I get scared when I feel sick, and much is self-induced. Felt very good all day. Vision graded 3+ on my 5-point scale. Weird feelings in my face and eye. Lots of drainage. Took five enzymes." These were my medical notes.

Our intentions here are to go to Steve's party, then meander around the countryside for a few days. In this place in the Lake Country, there are stone circles that no one but residents knows about. On an earlier visit I had been to a grove of yew trees and felt the urgency to visit them again, which we do the day after our arrival. After many wrong turns and bad directions, we arrive at a small cluster of hills with water flowing into a valley. Judy and I climb up, avoiding sheep turds and thistles. My ancestors worshiped the trees, this I know. This is Viking territory; the towns and streets are name memories of their language.

Some of the yews are at least five thousand years old. They grow in a unique way: the insides die off and shed pieces, they become hollow chapels, and the drooping branches create new trees. The shades of brown, yellow, orange, and red blend into a celestial visual harmony. I crawl inside one and know that I'm home. From inside a younger tree, I take dead pieces—each to represent what is no longer needed in my life—like plucking motes from the eye. My vision is really less distracting, if not better. It might be the light. I navigate the difficult, hilly terrain quite well, even with impaired depth perception.

The eye, again, seemed inconsequential in this sacred setting. I cried. Judy held me and whispered, "You don't always have to be brave." This time I was not being brave, I told her, but feeling the joy of connection. Another level of healing had just occurred.

———◇———

Medium sleep. No dreams—up until one o'clock the next morning. Wake achy but OK and feeling myself, which means my body feels as if it belongs to me—old familiar me and not some sick, cranky person. Eye feels snotty, with much drainage when I try to look out of it. I have learned about Steve's health episodes, which sound similar to ones I've had. He has head pain, disassociates, and has visions. This process acts like a cerebral bleed.

Steve relates another dream of me. I am spinning, dancing back and forth away from and toward a light near my feet. All around is dark. My long hair is swirling. He found himself wanting me to move toward the light. I make an attempt to redream this on a following night but cannot.

———◇———

Today, September 28, the eye felt normal. I felt entirely normal. We had lunch with Christopher and Pat Pilkington, the founders of the Bristol Cancer Center. May their praises someday be universally sung. Pat hugged me and said, "If you need us, call. Oceans do not matter." Just these past few months, she and Christopher had the honor of caring for Penny Brohn. Penny was the cofounder of the center and a marvel at repeatedly recovering from the worst sorts of cancers and their spread. She was also very beautiful and proud. The last few weeks of her life, she allowed Pat to wash her hair, bathe her, and take care of her in every way. After telling me about Penny, Pat looked over me and gasped, "But you have such a big angel with you. I see him." I also know that to be true. Pat has a very personal relationship with the angels, as does Christopher, a vicar in the Anglican Church.

At another "girls-only" dinner, we spoke of Ginny Hine again. I had put a rock she gave me into my medicine box for this trip. I need to find her. How many times have I written that? Jeannie, Judy, and I spoke of the "rock" consciousness as very low vibrational levels of energy. I've been systematically, consistently lowering my vibrational levels. Normally they are high (or so people tell me who seem to know about such things), and I zing around pretty tightly wired. People still see them as high. I don't. There has been something about being at home, in Santa Fe, doing what I'm trying to do, that makes me attempt to lower my vibrational levels, sleep, and leave. Is this what happens? Do we just run down like a battery-powered duck?

Judy thinks the Eye Thing has shrunk. I can't tell but had no sensations from it yesterday.

◇

Now we must travel to Durham Castle to teach, the alleged purpose of our trip. I have been to Durham Castle before, and it, too, is one of my favorite places on the planet. Steve and Jeannie allow us to stay in the castle in the Chaplain's Suite—a special privilege because there are only two suites in the castle proper. The castle is about eleventh-century, but with older and newer additions. The oldest is the Norman Chapel, underground and only recently discovered. Our first night in the castle is damp and cold but thrilling. I have what I call garbage dreams, probably of little significance, but still of houses and our yard. I am returning home; Carol, the gardener, is there. I'm trying to find the lavender plants I brought for her from Glastonbury.

Then I dream I am driving with some outlandish-looking woman to a workshop in California. We are on a "Stephen King" kind of road. A restaurant owner says I must "trade down" my car. It would be dangerous to be on the road with the one I have, since, I am, he said, a "university blonde." The road is very disorienting: it feels as if you're going backward. I look at a map and decide to go anyway. Dream ends. I am eating from a plate of nuts. Well, I am a "university blond" (although I can't say the phrase had ever entered my head before) and I am on a strange road, and we'll just leave the nut thing alone.

As I write, I am achy from the cold castle but normal at the core level. For the last three days, I realize that my quick wit ("rapier," Steve calls it) is back. I haven't been funny for some time.

Judy and I are going to do shamanic drumming in the old Norman Chapel at midnight during the conference. It does, needless to say, raise the spirits. When I planned the timing, I was remembering that it is at midnight when change most often is provoked and the barriers between the natural and supernatural are porous. I forgot how tired people would be after long days of conferencing and a heavy British dinner followed by dances with people from Findhorn. Oh well. Altered state of consciousness is guaranteed.

The four days in Durham could be a book unto themselves. The history, the burial of the Celtic saint Cuthbert, the miracles, the pilgrimages, and the wars are the stories of which movies are made.

I was caught in an ancient healing vortex, and as happened during the time with Michael Harner, I moved out of my body into another space and have only fragmentary memories. Steve and Jeannie planned a healing ritual for me. Steve and I have a primordial, bonded, old contract. Maybe I'm making this up, but it seems correct that some lifetimes I am his healer, and others, he is mine. We would do anything for each other. I remembered this as Judy and I went to their suite.

They placed nineteen candles around me. Prayers and invocations were given as the candles burned. Steve had visions. I had been in his dreams for more than a month, and his dreams of me had intensified over the past week. Steve gave me much information, and I can relate a little. He saw me as an eight-year-old girl, on a bed with a plaid blanket. I had obviously been crying for a long time. It seemed important for me to remember what this was about. It had to do with my vision, the rest of my life.

He anointed me with waters from Lourdes. He touched my eyes. Again, he, like Michael, focused on the right, or "good," eye. I quit questioning this. He had awakened that morning with the idea that I needed a sword for protection and went to the village to find one. He came back with a slice of white crystal. This was placed in my hand. At the end of the ceremony, he wrapped up the candles, the bottle of water, and the crystal in a silk purple scarf and then in his black shirt.

These gifts went home with me, and I continued to use them. Each day, after arriving home, I lit one of the nineteen candles. They were sturdy tea lights and had lots of life left in them. Now I must remember that nineteen has been *the* number. It was integral to Steve's first dreams as well as to my continued meditation, and it was only weeks later, on the nineteenth of November, that my eye began to explode and I held on for dear life.

It was during the drumming that Judy and I did in the Norman Chapel that Steve had even more powerful visions. On the first night of drumming (before the healing ritual I described above), Steve had an extraordinarily painful experience. As we drummed, I watched with alarm as he made sudden eye contact with me. He'd seen something frightful, like a ghost. He ran and then crouched by the old altar. In one vision he saw me being attacked, by a head with only one eye and with large teeth. It said, "I will be the grief of her." I am reminded of the "elementals," as they are called in some metaphysical beliefs. They are pure evil and have no intentions to speak of, like a hex or curse; they are things that fly around and from which there is little protection. Often they are associated with cancer, a friend who has studied this has told me. Primal evil, if you can imagine that, is the worst kind because there is no negotiation, no control.

After the drumming Judy and I sat quietly until people left. The drumming was powerful: some cried; others remained suspended in space and needed help coming back to ground. When most had gone, Steve came to the bench where I was sitting and encircled me with his legs and arms. Every mortal, man or woman, who has laid eyes on Steve falls in love, and I was no exception. Sitting between his legs was quite wonderful, and I felt a stirring of sensuality that had been absent from my life for far too long. We stayed that way, rocking gently, for maybe ten or fifteen minutes. I smelled him: his aroma was not like any other. I'm glad that he wrapped the nineteen candles in his black T-shirt after the healing ceremony: it is now part and parcel of my medicine bundle. There is much of Steve around me. I wear an amulet—a mysterious stone—that he wore for many years. The bag containing it must have been blue velvet at one time. I have to remember to return it to him soon.

I'm still walking in Steve's dreams, and he surely wants some peaceful sleep. On the very last hour of the last day of the conference, Judy and I go out to the courtyard to say good-bye to him and Jeannie. It is raining still—has not stopped since we landed. Under our umbrellas, Steve says, "I found a protection for you last night during the drumming. It was a wild man, wearing feathers. He painted your body for protection."

"Who is he, or what is he?"

"I don't know. I've never seen him before. When you see it, you will know he is there for you."

I didn't see it first, but Steve did—the next week in Glastonbury, of all places. He saw a poster depicting what had been painted on my body. The symbol turned out to be a rune—one of the ancient Nordic letters used for divination and communication. It was algiz, the rune of protection and defense. This rune also symbolizes preservation in the face of adversity. Algiz serves as a mirror for the inner self and is concerned with controlling emotions so as not to collapse into the highs and lows and become a victim of circumstance. Steve later sends me material on this rune. It is represented by the swan. It is said that he carries the talent of enhancing one's hearing and eyesight. Algiz is especially linked with the hamingja, the protective spirit-woman who accompanies individuals on the path toward the divine self. The oracular meaning (according to the book *The Rune Mysteries*) is protection; it reveals a powerful, protective energy that is making itself felt in one's life. It predicts a fortunate influence.

Steve related one more dream: one of the nineteen gold ropes or ribbons had dropped away. He seemed to think it was a good omen.

We left the next day to go back to the United States. I knew that several more levels of my self had been touched and healed. And it wasn't just from ceremony. Judy Ostrow is a medicine woman in several senses of the term, including as an everyday-type healer, who uses regular activities as medicine. One morning, for example, she said, "I'm going to dry your hair."

"What do you mean, dry my hair?"

"Haven't you ever had anyone but a hairdresser do that?"

No, I hadn't, but Judy does things like that. She gave me a foot massage in Glastonbury just for the heck of it. It was *her* feet that were hurting, I think. I get squirrelly when people do such things for me. She knows that.

Judy and I laughed like hyenas, and that, too, was medicine. One morning one of the conference assistants (a very young, sweet man) came to our door. Judy had just teased her hair and it was standing up as if she'd been electrocuted, and I was staggering around with coffee cup in hand, six hot curlers in my hair, and my robe gaping open to reveal the awful truth. The dear young man looked at us, gulped, decided he had the wrong address, and left like a streak of greased lightning. We laughed; I fell down laughing, kicking my feet up in the air; our sides ached. Judy said, "Jeanne, I haven't seen you do that for two years." True, I hadn't really laughed for at least that long. Later we apologized to the young fellow, who replied, "That's all right. I have four sisters. I've seen these things." We were redeemed.

We also did things that were very silly for ladies of our age and station. In England they have Cadbury chocolate machines. Cadbury is *not* Snickers. Cadbury is something to die for—chocolate that, they say, is better than sex. Around midnight we would get the cravings. "Judy," says I, "this is addiction."

"I know. Let's go."

"It's still raining."

"Roll up your pajama pants, put on your raincoat, and let's head out." So we spirit ourselves past the minions of the castle and make a beeline for the machines.

Healing times. I am truly sorry that Frank, once again, missed major turning points on this journey. But he did. He was invited repeatedly and had declined.

On the second of October, Jim Lake sent me a wonderful CD and images: "In the mornings I sometimes imagine your face until I can capture your image perfectly. Then I imagine soft, warm light suffusing your head and eyes, bringing relief—perhaps white-blue light that can help make up for the light you cannot take in from the world."

Christa, a woman of the Church who was in one of our trainings, always manages to send just the perfect messages at the right times:

> Not a day goes by that I don't think about you and "set sacred intention." I don't know what it means to "pray for" anything, but I somehow I think that whatever it is that I hold lovingly in my heart is taken up into the abiding, loving Presence of the universe. I treasure the woman that you are and the woman I continually see emerging—moving ever closer to that wholeness that surrounds us. My love and care also to Frank. I know that whenever suffering comes to one we love, it comes to the other, also. In fact, in the love you share, the lines between "other" and the self become so blurred. What exquisite beauty! What gift! Dearest One, be assured of continued loving care.

When I arrived home, these treasures would await me.

Days of Reckoning

{October 3}

ON THE WAY HOME I wrote more self-reflections. Getting to be the same old boring shit, but the writing, obsessive or not, preserves sanity somehow. I wrote:

> I do hope that Frank is not sick, as he usually is when I come home. I feel so desperately in need of more skills, more something. I wish we could be lovers again.
>
> What terrible things these are to write after a pilgrimage. If only he had been there. Why is he choosing to miss the divine parts of this journey and just getting the butt end, which is me dragging around the house worrying about several million things?

There are other things I must change when I get home. The way I earn a living, for one thing. How many more papers must I read? I need to open up my vision, as I did when I became the eight-year-old princess. (Funny, Steve refers to me always as "the princess," but he doesn't know about that part of my life. It must still show.) Let me pretend there is a future, and this is what it could be like:

- Each daily activity is an act of meditation.
- I go to sleep in peace and wake up excited.
- Work is creative.
- At least once a week, I laugh until I fall down.
- Animals and flowers are everywhere.

- The kids are making their lives work.
- Girlfriends.
- Slow mornings, time for coffee, books, walks for fun.
- Evenings. Hmmm—these are difficult. Will take some more thought.
- People around me every day.

Dark Weeks

{October 4}

HOMECOMING WAS A black time. As the retina detached fully, vision was lost. All the decisions were right back in my face. The fun times were over. I'd much rather dabble about in the spiritual realm, where there is some sense of eternity and a bigger picture, than return to modern medicine, which, it seems, is rejecting me as I am rejecting it.

The office of Eye Doc (E.D.) had already resolved any ambivalence I might have had about hiring its services. An office assistant had called and left a message on my answering machine telling me they'd scheduled me to see someone—probably the oncologist—at a time when I wasn't even in the country. I needed more tests, and I needed to have them done there. Seems the instructions had changed again. When I had first been scheduled back in September, I was asked to have the tests done in Santa Fe and bring the reports with me. Now that would not be possible. The outgoing message on my answering machine had clearly specified that no messages should be left under any circumstances—that I was traveling and would not be checking my machine and that anyone needing to reach me in an emergency should call my husband. The assistant from E.D.'s office had left a message anyway. It was only a fluke that Frank found it.

I promptly canceled medical diagnostic workups for the "bomb" treatment in self-defense. In fairness, I never gave a full explanation of why. I wrote a letter but didn't mail it. Later someone on E.D.'s staff called and told Frank that the office now had a patient coordinator and if I was interested in coming back, I would be welcomed. But if an organization can't get its act together to schedule appointments and isn't humane enough to ask rather than tell me when to come in for appointments at facilities a considerable distance away, what would make me trust its people to poke around in my eye?

This information, most of which I got while in England, prompted me to compose a list of questions to be faxed for second opinions. I do not expect free services; I offer to pay for a telephone consultation. If this second level of doctors won't answer these questions, I'm not likely to allow them to touch me either. I should have formulated these questions long before. I always advise my patients to do it. But you just can't get around to everything. Some of my questions were simple, like "How many patients with this problem have you treated?" Some were not so simple, like "What role do you believe the patient can play in the healing process?"

Not one of the second-opinion docs would answer a single question. They insisted on seeing me first. I don't get it. If my diagnosis is cut-and-dried, and they have only two treatment options (poke it out or burn it), answering these questions should be no problem. I did speak with the second- and third-opinion docs, briefly, and they seemed genuinely interested. None of these docs is soliciting patients; they have plenty already, I have been assured. In a reasonably compassionate way, I was told I should just have my eye removed, because that is what would eventually happen anyway.

The time between my homecoming from England and my departure for Germany on November 3 was troublesome, although my healing resources, the prayers and supportive network, were still in full swing. The pressure to do something before it is too late is intensifying. My mother is the biggest factor here, and one that must soon be reckoned with. But I, too, am falling under the spell of Western medical dogma, which holds that I must radically destroy the eye—or else. "Or else *what?*" I have to ask myself. I begin to wonder whether what I am doing—which is to change my whole life, examine the very nature of reality, alter my chemistry—counts as doing nothing.

I have to keep reminding myself that I can read, I know the data. The treatment is barbaric, almost guaranteed to kill an eye. Not one of the many eye docs noted that I work with my eyes, that my physical appearance is part of my livelihood, and that my other eye, if uncorrected, is considered legally blind. Medical treatment can only provide local control, at best. What kills you isn't the ocular melanoma; it's the metastasis. And treatment is statistically likely to be followed by metastasis, at least according to some studies that no one wants to talk about anymore merely because they are not considered sufficiently recent.

———◇———

In the midst of all this decision making about medical treatment, Frank and I spent a day meditating together in order to get the relationship dragons to settle down. I think it was around October 9. We tried to be in a place of emotional stillness, but I paced the floor, took a reading on Frank, changed the music, cooked a little soup from garden veggies, and was left exhausted for about four days.

We tried to discuss our fears. I decided my primary fear was not finishing my business, doing what I was supposed to do this lifetime, because it did not feel complete. During this day of reckoning, Frank said his biggest fear was losing himself during my healing process and set his boundaries once and for all: he could provide only twelve weeks. I do not know how he calculated this—whether it was on an annual basis or what. Did it include vacations? Were we supposed to keep a debit and credit system? How much had been used up already? The details were never addressed, but I would rather drown myself than ask for time. The discussion hung like crepe around us.

I am, as I said, fearful of not finishing my business here, afraid of leaving loves unloved, children unmothered, work incomplete because of pain and inertia. I am afraid of disappointing all those who see me as some kind of exemplar for how a woman can survive in a difficult professional world. Thoughts of a lingering death in which I have to endure the hysteria of others frighten me, as does the prospect of not passing with honor. Most of all, I think I have been hibernating for a long time and fear I will not live long enough to wake up.

———◇———

During this period I have to face the *mother* problem. I am a phantom daughter. My mother knows little about me. I don't tell her how I earn a living nor how I spend my quiet hours nor my huge joys or my failures. I don't lie; I just don't talk. My brothers talk more, lie a little, but they live close by, and she can look into their lives with greater ease. She is proud of me, and my books are about the only ones in her house.

Two years ago we asked Mom and her husband, Will, whether they would like to live in our home for a month while we went to Europe. It meant that she spent an unprecedented length of time around my things. Our home is magnificent, and Santa Fe is a tourist delight, so of course, they agreed. The major caretaker responsibility would have been the two birds, which disappeared off the front porch the day we left.

Frank came home from Europe before I did and found that the house, especially the kitchen, had been rearranged.

"Your things," Mom said, "are in the wrong place."

Now she has an unruly, peculiar daughter, whose things are not in the right place, maybe dying because she won't do "the right thing." I finally ask what she considers the right thing, getting my eye burned out or cut out. I explain the consequences of each. But meanwhile, another thread of thought plagues me. Yes, something *did* happen when I was eight years old. Steve Wright and the medical intuitive both noted it as profoundly associated with my illness and healing. Miriam Goldberg and Steve had visions of me at about that age on a bed with a dark spread, quiet, not happy, apparently having been crying. Coincidence?

I must go back, painfully, to this time. For one thing I was having difficulty reading the blackboard in school. They took me to the eye doctor and found that my vision was about 20/400 in both eyes. Not only couldn't I see the leaves; I couldn't even see the trees.

No one alive can help me recapture the memories. My mother has even forgotten places where we lived when I was six or seven. Our lives were a series of migrations. I had to get out old report cards to prove to her that we were in Oregon, for instance. "We never lived there," she said. The report cards, which were pretty specific, said we had. My aunt, who is only twelve years older than I am, has dim memories of my grandparents' traveling to get us kids and finding there was no food in the house.

Here's what I think. The world had just gotten awful by then. I had been the cherished firstborn in a large family during World War II—a symbol of "life goes on." Even my uncles wrote me cards from the battlefields, which I still have, and sent me gifts and mementos from wherever they were. I looked like a little princess (more like Shirley Temple after they messed up my hair with electric curlers and a very smelly perm) and must have believed that I was one. My grandmother was always with me and, I suspect, did most of the mothering because my mother always worked.

Grandma remains forever in my heart, and I think—no, I know—that she saved my life, not only by spiriting me away when I was in danger but by teaching me to love flowers, poetry, and myself. We listened to the soaps every day, and then—in what must surely have been a demonstration of unconditional love—she would sit quietly with her hands folded while I banged on the piano.

Out of this a wildflower was nurtured—if indeed, wildflowers can be cultivated to any extent. She and I would go out into the mountains and meadows while Granddad fished for trout, and we would dig up the beautiful columbines and other flowers whose names I didn't know and take them to her garden. "They don't transplant well, you know. They are best left to their own devices." I decided then and there that I was a wildflower.

We were all casualties of the war. My father refused to look at me or hold me, I was later told. My mother said she didn't recognize him: he'd gotten crazy and slept with a gun. Nearly killed her a couple of times. Too much war, too many dead boys around him. He was only twenty-two when he first saw action. He got addicted to many things: alcohol, cigarettes, and intensity. He volunteered for the Korean War and mercifully left us again when I was eight.

I had to reinvent myself, so I went back to being a princess. I secretly practiced holding my hands daintily, waving that little stiff wave, curtseying, doing princess things. I tied ribbons crisscross around my shoes and legs because it looked like the illustration of a princess in one of my fairy-tale books. I lied and told my fellow third graders that my grandparents were rich. I said my real name was Katinka van Winkle, which sounded quite royal enough. We lived in the tenements—Stewart Homes (government-sponsored and income-regulated)—so it was hard to pull off the image for long. I got busted and never did much lying after that.

At some financial sacrifice, I'm sure, I was given one dollar a week—enough for a bus into town and a ballet lesson, so in addition to being a princess, I was going to become a famous dancer.

At night I spent hours clearly imaging scenes over and over again. I had married a dentist (dentists being about the only professionals I was aware of) and had beautiful clothes dripping with lace. My life was perfect—at least, in this theater of my imagination.

But what else must I remember? All of a sudden, I got smart again when I was eight and made the best grades in class. I read voraciously, even cereal boxes and telephone books. My third-grade teacher convinced Mom that I had some talent and sold her a *World Book Encyclopedia* set on a monthly payment plan. I read every entry from A to Z and then would start over again. I couldn't sleep in those days, either. Mom said, "You just think too much. That's why you can't ever sleep."

She worked steadily until her husband got back from the next war, when I was eleven, and the baby-sitters usually took the boys and left me alone. Benign neglect characterized my upbringing as it has my marriage, and I'm glad. There were few restraints on what I did or thought because no one paid much attention.

I read the Bible over and over and prayed a lot. Mostly, during the third grade, I prayed that my boobs wouldn't get any bigger and that, if they did, I would not have to strip naked and take showers during gym class—which is what the fourth graders did. I can never remember having prayed with such intensity. It worked: the gym was under construction, and we did not have physical education that year. My boobs kept getting bigger, though.

I have to backtrack a bit and interject another piece of information here, and whether it has to do with magic or prayer is really not essential to the story. During our time in California (I must have been five or six then, because I started first grade), Mom went to work to supplement our income. We lived in temporary buildings that had been constructed to house troops being trained at Fort Ord. (The fact that those buildings are still standing says something about military construction.)

We were placed in the care of a woman who had a twelve-year-old daughter. The woman took the boys off during the day (to her mother's in Seaside, I believe). The daughter took care of me, if it could be called that. She was practicing black witchcraft, or something close to it. She was conversant with symbols, ceremonies, and ideas that I find rather strange for someone her age, unless it was a familial tradition. Usually the afternoon would start with her holding a butcher knife to my neck, threatening to kill me if I ever told anyone. I believed her and didn't. I begged my mother not to leave me with her but didn't dare tell her why. There was no question in my mind then (nor is there now) that she was dangerous. Her name is Cynthia Woods. I've been looking for her for half a century or so.

Cynthia tied me up out in the fields behind Fort Ord and made me go into holes that she said were snake pits. In the playground she would put a "spell" on things like bolts, then tell me they were red-hot and poke me with them. I can't remember whether I blistered, but it is certainly possible, given what we now know about hypnosis. At her grandparents' house in Seaside, Cynthia had a witchy, nasty environment in an unused chicken coop where she did her magic. I can still smell it. Often she sent me off to talk to the cats, probably when she was tired of messing with me. In one of my discussions with the cats, I expressed in no uncertain terms that I wanted Cynthia to stop what she was doing to me and asked whether they would help. I do not remember asking that any harm come to her, but I may have. They, or something, did help—and within days.

Her grandparents burned leaves and garbage, and Cynthia would always dance around the fire barefoot, which gives you some idea of how unusual the girl was. This time, after my little conversation with the cats, when she danced around in the ashes, there were still live embers, unbeknownst to her. The next day when I was dropped off at her house, Cynthia had her feet propped up and bandaged (must have been second-degree burns, at least), and she was out of commission for the rest of the summer. I was free. I never told my mom about Cynthia until we moved and I knew I would be safe. So began my history with the occult, prayer, and the imagination.

Inventing a life out of paltry means, limited experience, an unbridled imagination, and a need for survival—that's what I did. Now I have the opportunity to do it again. Do I have the same skills? The same strength? The Life Force on my side? When you are only eight, you have to get really creative and find totally novel solutions, just because you haven't been around for long or done much. But you also don't have as much baggage to jettison as you do later on. This year would need to be one not just of remembering but also of mercilessly stripping down, getting close to the bone to see what was essential, redeemable, and pure. There would need to be less of me before there could be more—that was becoming all too obvious.

I have to think about the mother thing. She's sending and bringing me gifts, calling and E-mailing constantly. Always the same questions, the need to have me answer in a way that would reassure her of my survival. I understand, but I cannot comply nor bring myself to tell lies, even little white ones. She doesn't approve of me, my lifestyle in which things are in the wrong place, or my treatment decisions. She continues to pressure me until I can stand it no longer. I remember last year during my own daughter's crisis, when the roles were reversed and I felt miserably inept and very critical of her lifestyle. My daughter had every reason not to want me around either, but she never said so.

The information that I gain by revisiting the eight-year-old girl sparks the need to stop the mothering pattern and to remember the magic of survival. I had to reexamine that time to remember what survival is all about and how I got through the rough spots, went from lonely and homely to valedictorian and head cheerleader.

———◇———

Let's get out of my ancient past for a moment. On October 17 Stanley Krippner, my colleague and old friend, was near Rio de Janeiro doing a ceremony. He wrote:

> A shaman and I went into the woods and built a sacred fire. We conducted a three-hour ritual on your behalf, calling upon the elements of fire, water, wind, earth, metal, and wood—all on behalf of your healing. It was a wonderful interaction between our intent and various surprises that nature had in store for us, just like a conversation—with sudden flares of the fire to punctuate my comments about you and sudden gusts of wind when we wanted to send prayers in your direction. So add another one on to the loving efforts made in your behalf.

I wrote back:

I am so very, very touched about the ceremony. I feel so undeserv-
ing, privileged, and stunned. That Sunday was a difficult day for
me. I had spiral flashes of light in that eye—golden light—and half
circles of light at the lower part of the eye. I then lost most of what
little vision I had left. I called my transpersonal eye doctor (August
Reader), and he said it could be a good thing, actually. It might
mean more of an inflammatory response. Stanley, you are so good
to me. I just love you.

Jeanne

And Stanley responded:

Actually, when we built the fire, we directed the flames toward
burning out the cancer in your retina. So your report takes on new
meaning!

Love,
Stan

———◇———

One morning about a week later my mother and Will "dropped in" on
me. Auuugh! You don't exactly drop in on someone who lives in another state. At least I was up and had been to the grocery store and was
not in my usual slovenly, enrobed, early-morning state of desperately
wanting to sleep through the whole nightmare. Those were the days
when I was not feeling well, probably from fear and my self-prescribed
immune-stimulation regimen, and slept as much as I could simply to
make the time pass.

"I just had to see you with my own eyes. We'll only stay for a while
and take you to lunch." I had to stop the pattern. I told her that her
mothering was overwhelming me right now and that I needed some
space from it. I was being suffocated by demands to be something I
was not.

I also asked about the events of the unspoken-of years and described,
in vivid detail, some of the few scenes that I could remember.

Mom had been on overdrive when I was eight, working to support
us three kids, and her amnesia regarding the earlier years was worse

than mine. Maybe the precise details of what happened didn't matter so much as the fact that we all got through it with a sense of humor (my brothers are pretty funny as well).

I told Mom I needed to recapture some of the memories myself. When big chunks disappear from your life, when you can't distinguish between dream houses and places you've really lived, it gets disturbing, and it must be for her, too. And I told her, "I am fighting for my life by trying to understand my life. Something happened when I was young that I need to know about. It will give me strength for healing."

They left quickly. The calls stopped. Mom would phone Frank at work instead for a status report. She and Will blamed my failure to be cured on the idea that I was not seeing real doctors but going to social workers in the mountains, and all they did was dig up dirt from your childhood so you could blame ugly things on your family. It was an interesting misperception, not at all true, but I didn't know how to correct it.

Mom still backslides now and then, and so do I. Three times one week she called to ask whether I was still doing the mistletoe. She's trying, though. She asked me whether I wanted the name of a doctor in California who uses herbs for cancer. "No, Mom, I'm full of herbs, but thanks anyway." I almost wish one of my brothers would get into some kind of trouble to take her mind off me for a while.

I should have followed my original plan—and not told her I was sick until three days after my death. Oh, but that would have left unfinished business, and the lingering ghost of my father reminds me that I must finish business, and do it with honor. Mom is from another generation—no, another world. I'm the one who will come to some healing terms with my life, not her.

Probably around the twenty-fifth of October, when I was in deep decision time, I wrote in my journal a letter to Frank:

> Frank:
> What a day. Please take my ego out of what I am going to write. I know I am a collective product, but that brings me no less pain. We have to honor bodies and spirits in different ways. To take out an eye or a breast or a prostate gland is a sacred act and a violation of humanity. We are killing parts of bodies and bodies as well. You

and I must somehow be part of the cure. I hate that it has to be on my own fabulous, healthy, beautiful body. But where else? Excuse me! And where else than on your generous, tender nature?

Obviously someone has tried to get me to poke out my eye again. I'm trying to be militant and brave and "see" the larger picture. A mission for humanity. I can do anything if it's going to be that—get maimed, suffer martyrdom, you name it. Senseless agony is torture of the worst sort. Why doesn't the Great One tell me what this is all about? What do those fucking, pardon my French, spirits want of me? Other people hear voices, get messages, and have revelations. Some of my best sources just do a few "sacred plants" and their god shows up. Unfortunately I guess that will not be my path; it's just life instead. I can't see where I'm going, as on the nosebleed night of the Vision Quest, but maybe if I pay attention, my soft-soled shoes will find the way.

Cards, E-mails, and support continue to roll in and buoy me up. I am feeling dead as a doornail and just move from chair to chair or bed to bed. Rain Borden supports my need to be still: "If living this has been a paralysis, maybe that's absolutely perfect for you right now, Jeanne. Maybe you just need some real 'stillness' to let the deep inner movements of Psyche have all the energy necessary to do her work. You are deeply loved, and all the angels are hard at work on your behalf. Be still as long as you need to be. You'll know when the time for a cycle of motion comes again."

I was, in the meantime, working myself up to facing the possibility of radiation, got into a diagnostic/treatment stream again, and the story from August and September repeated itself. I balked at the orders left on my answering machine and the surprises and was told by a member of an office staff that I was not being cooperative and not acting in the best interests of my own health. I got pissed but held my tongue—a rarity, of course.

I am no doubt a royal pain in the butt, but it is my eye and its treatment has serious consequences for my life, including whether I might become a bag lady if I could no longer see to read or write. These ideas do cross your mind, especially if you don't have a decent pension plan or much disability insurance. Many of my generation figured we'd have no need for such things because we (1) were never going to quit work or (2) would just suddenly drop dead.

More messages from medical offices are left on an answering machine that is not located where I am, telling me to show up for tests fifteen hundred miles away at a specified time, very soon, but providing no clue as to what the tests would be for. Canceled. The omens are not boding well, and thus far only the omens, dreams, and intuition have been consistent and reliable.

The antidotes for the confusion and terror were the notes, calls, E-mails, and gifts that arrived daily. From Sandy Baumann, a woman who had been in several of my training programs, I received a cloth saturated with tears from a crying Madonna in an Orthodox monastery in Blanco, Texas. When she weeps, the monks collect the tears, and they are often associated with miracles. Thanks to Sandy and others, my own home is becoming a healing shrine, and I expect lines of tourists to start forming any day to bear witness to one of the larger and more eclectic collections of sacred artifacts.

Meanwhile, Jean Bolen called to check in. She has written many books on healing, my current favorite being the very quotable *Close to the Bone*—about health, meaning, life, and death, which were very close to my bones just then. She told me about Mark Rennecker, who is, in my estimation, the physician of the future. He is a medical detective, an M.D. who no longer practices medicine but does "curbside" consultation. He researches strange cases. He talks to doctors, and they tell him things they won't tell patients. He is clearly well versed on both the mainstream and the alternative scene. He agreed to take my "case" and do some digging around. He became about the only one I trusted with my health because my health is his only interest—not any particular treatment.

Mark told me about his father, a psychotherapist who was diagnosed with (I think) a rare tumor of the parotid (the salivary gland located near the base of the ear). The only option offered to his father was to have the tumor removed, which meant he would also lose muscle control over half his face. He could not imagine himself practicing psychotherapy while drooling. His dad lived in New York and was a friend of Larry LeShan's. So he went to a very young doctor at Travis Air Force Base (none other than my buddy Carl Simonton) and began using imagery. Mark's dad convinced his doctor to allow him to try to shrink the tumor a little so that the surgery would not be so devastating. It worked. As Mark told me this, I was not sure whether he knew of my connection with either Carl or Larry.

———◇———

After a rugged couple of weeks, there occurred a remarkable day in this process of medicine practiced by default and intuition. One by one, until November 2, my options had been orchestrated not by me but by that Big Hand, and I didn't even know it. When there are no promises of health and the only guarantee is that you will lose a precious part of yourself, treatment decisions are anguishing. I remained at a loss for words, or even for a metaphor or an analogy, to express just what kind of horror this presents. This period of uncertainty was far worse than the weeks after the diagnosis, when I had been cocooned by shock, busy every waking hour searching out treatment options, doing my time-consuming kill-or-cure routine, and being the grateful recipient of so much tenderness. I was felled by the propaganda that I was risking my life by not presenting myself for medical treatment.

I had been on-again, off-again about the radioactive plaque and finally, after looking at the procedure in a textbook one more time, decided I could not undergo this surgery—some voice deep inside screamed "No!" Something not so deep prompted me with what I knew for sure: I could not survive two general anesthesias in a short period of time. I honestly did try to get with the program on this treatment. A few of the girlfriends and I were once again going to make the best of it: we would sequester ourselves—with the others suitably out of range of radioactive me, of course—and write a book we'd been planning about our unusual mothers, who deserved a tribute.

Every cell in my body rebelled, not only against the plaque therapy (which I continued to misspell as "plague therapy") but against the proton radiation and eye removal. I cried, ranted, and completely forgot how to contact my spiritual and intuitive resources but did call upon my human resources. Whining like a sick cat, I asked about the decision-making processes they used in evaluating radical medical treatment. Always the answer involved some element of trust. I remembered my own lectures about faith and trust as essential ingredients in all successful treatment, and maybe these were more important than the therapy itself. If you look at the history of medicine, and all the outrageous treatments inflicted on the species, and the fact that some people do get well even if they are purged, bled, and burned, you just have to conclude that what accounts for a cure is what goes on between the ears and not the treatment per se. Trust and faith were not going on between my ears.

A nurse friend called the day before I left for Mo's. She had just spoken about my situation with her husband, an oncologist, who obviously had no stake in my treatment. He said, "She has nothing to gain by aggressive treatment and everything to lose—her eye, her appearance, and maybe her health. You don't die from ocular melanoma, you die from its metastasis—and fast—and there is no treatment. Sometimes it doesn't metastasize for thirty years, sometimes never, whether it is treated or not." I knew all this, but I needed to hear it one more time from an objective source. I realized that I might already have micrometastasis and that the best treatment was what I was doing—trying to take care of myself and stimulate my immune system in the best possible way.

So Mo, one more time, agrees to go with me into the dreaded medical system, as a steadfast accomplice who knows when to listen and when to speak with a direct and sane voice. I had shown her the pictures of the plaque surgery, and she said, "That's just because they don't know what else to do." As usual, she evaluates my decisions with honesty and this time agrees with me (which she does not always do, I might add). Because of the experience with her daughter, Mo understands scary cancer treatment that holds little promise. In her nononsense way, she says, "Dr. Good Doc isn't going to refuse to follow you if you don't do his treatment, and if he does, go find someone else to monitor the Thing." Why do I have to keep being reminded that I'm in charge here?

Mark knew that I was going to see Dr. Good Doc and said he was the best in the field. I explained to Mark my anguish about treatment decisions and told him that I could not, just yet, put myself on the table. Mark coached me on how to approach having a doctor monitor me while I tried "other things" to get the tumor to a manageable size. I memorized a couple of sentences about wanting careful scrutiny and monitoring. I was not to mention that I was trying to get rid of it with "alternatives," because that would probably result in my being pressured to get it treated right away. The "alternatives" might not do the trick either, but I needed to buy some time, needed to find something to trust. I called Mark twice while on Highway 101 to get reassurance on my way to Good Doc's office. If those huge bird-type guardian angels are really there, and they seem to be, they flew Mark my way or vice versa.

I got another sonogram that day. Good Doc said the Thing had grown. But we couldn't teli for sure. On a sonogram inflammatory activity can't be distinguished from a tumor: the whole thing simply looks like a spot. Regardless, the apparent size had moved beyond the far edge of what Good Doc would be comfortable in treating with the plaque. Might be too big even for the bomb. I then told him my plan, which was to use whatever I could to stimulate my immune system to see whether my own defenses could shrink it to a size that would be more manageable by treatment. I asked him whether he would be willing to monitor the tumor while I tried the alternatives. I held my breath, waiting for his answer. He replied, "It would be an honor. This is the only way medicine makes progress, by someone who is willing to try a different way." I told him that I knew it was immunoreactive, that I had spoken with immunologists. He flattered me by saying, "You know things I don't. I will respect that." I suspect, but do not know, that he was uncomfortable with my decisions nevertheless. I wrote him a long letter, explained what I was doing, sent him a review article on mistletoe, and told him if he was uncomfortable—ever—legally or otherwise, to let me know.

Germany: Same Time, Next Year

{November 3}

I AM WRITING on the airplane to Munich. It is the annual trek to Zist, a retreat in Bavaria, to teach with Carl Simonton. This time I'm wondering whether my newly diagnosed status will have an impact on teaching these would-be cancer counselors. Most of them in the training now are physicians and health-care practitioners who have great, open hearts and a desire to be the healers they were meant to be. I vow to watch my diet a little better. Someone told me melanoma feeds on sugar. (Carl said, "Nonsense. All cells feed on sugar. If you're worried about it, don't eat it.")

Having been negligent in my journaling, I try to catch up on the long flight, writing, "This is the day I need to begin writing to save my life and record my life. Hope I have enough paper! I have been too frozen in fear to think, much less read or write. Now I have no excuses."

It was with a lighter heart than usual that I boarded the plane on November 3. I figure my goal is to blaze a trail. And I must have courage, clarity, and commitment. Do I want to stay alive? Yes and no. At least now I say, "Yes, maybe." We're making progress here. In May I would have said, "No." Life had given me a terrible hit. Now I am out on the edge, so there is nothing much more to dread or fear. All that remains is curiosity. What is this piece of life about? I would like to have the Thing go into remission and, since I am such a public figure, have a story that increases my kindness and gentleness to people who are sick

150

and afraid. I don't have a clear fix on this for me—especially since I am a skeptic at heart and a mystic by desire. I am not my body, but it does command my moments of attention. I, the alleged visionary, am going blind. How perfect.

Maureen O'Hara, the president of Saybrook Graduate School, where I teach, said something about the fate of master teachers who need more to teach: life leads them on to more material. Although it is nice that she thinks I am a master teacher, I could have done better with a few less obsessions and a little more vision.

Mo and I spoke of "blind fury" before I left. I guess I do have anger. Never had much time for it before, except in dreams. Yes, I probably am in a blind fury and need to work through it to clear my vision. God grant me the time and strength to do so. I have to hold my ground, stay trusting in something, not wallow in the darkness, and remember to finish my contract with life. I cannot self-destruct, must stay awake and truthful and faithful. And keep writing.

I have to be aware of the thousands of people who pray for my health, for a return of vision. I'm sure some also pray for my life. Not one has said that he or she intuits me as maimed or dead—but who would tell me that anyway? None of these people are in my body, however, and experiencing the progressive loss of sight, the strange sensations, the final disruption of most of the vision.

On the plane I continue to write:

> I must invent a new life—if I am to live, that is. This old life is now dead, tedious, hurtful, and adds nothing to the growth of humanity in even a small way. I'm taking up space. I continue to self-reflect, and as I write this, I am getting bored with myself again. I try to look honestly at who I am or was. Yes, I was smart, and very nice. And humble. (Ha-ha.) I was consumed and led by passion, and this must be rekindled. It was fired by romance in the early days, and that steered me down a life path. It kept me with Frank even during his difficult times in California. Many, many years ago, it connected me to Carl in a peculiar way. I never felt any physical attraction to him until I had a dream about a year after we met. Immediately, the next day, passion got added to our working relationship and sparked much of our creativity. Is this the end of physical passion? What a pity.

Again and again in this writing, I remind myself to be strong, not vulnerable or dependent—to remember the eight-year-old who re-invented herself.

About the vision. When my Vision returns, my vision will return. As of this writing I have no intention of sacrificing an eye, of all things. I will sacrifice my present view of the world for a new one. I need to wake up, renew my curiosity.

Now, as the hours go by, I come back to the Eye Thing. Days of meditation would be good. Light-filled days. Walking. Let the desired intention for my life be fulfilled. My imagery needs to be of gentleness, rest. My vision should rest. My writing should be done with softness. I can imagine the tumor dying gently, cell by cell. No inflammation, only softness, the retina gradually reattaching. But first, each cell drops off as I peel away layers, leaves, of what I cannot take forward. The Thing is a black substance condensed from the poisons of my own despair. When Vision returns, vision returns.

The process of imagery itself is not yet mythic, and I am back to biological imagery—imaging apoptosis, the natural death of cells. I cannot feed the process with despair, fear, and chemicals any longer. My eye actually feels tight and burny: a rush of something flows through it.

Am I stepping toward death or life? Both, of course; it is always both. The physical sentence just brings clarity. But all this needs to be addressed, as does the blind fury. Then I can move on.

I have to make difficult decisions about the company I currently keep. I, who want to be the beloved princess of the world, will have to keep certain people away until I can regroup. I do not need anyone around me right now who feeds on my vision, my ideas, or me. That does not mean a cessation of love or regard but merely that the doors between us be closed temporarily. Maybe permanently; I just can't tell. I simply need a period of reorganization.

On this day Martha Overton wrote a letter that I read when I got home:

> I've been praying for your eye since Margaret Christensen first told me. The day we went to Guadelupe Cathedral in Dallas to pray and Saint Lucy's picture appeared was one of the most amazing prayerful times I've experienced in quite a while. You were very close to

us even as we drove to Guadelupe, since Margaret showed me the healing images box she was creating for you. We were praying in the small chapel where so many prayers of the Hispanic faithful linger, and Margaret followed the downward gaze of Our Lady's eyes and Our Lady was looking at the picture of Saint Lucy on the floor propped against the wall! When we saw the "eyes" in the Saint Lucy's picture, we knew it was a holy moment and it was for your healing that she appeared. As Margaret secured the picture for you, Saint Lucy became our "spontaneous appearance" of love and support for you—blessed teacher and wise woman. I believe a "spontaneous remission" is already happening in your eye and my prayers continue for your complete healing. You are a tremendous influence in my life, and all you taught me at ITP [Institute of Transpersonal Psychology] resonates deep within me. One thought that I remember often from your 1994 Woman as Healer conference at Baylor is that "women need to write." That just comes up over and over as I remember the passion you had that day. You are incredibly gifted with wisdom and beauty, and may your time of healing bring you deep peace.

———◇———

Despite having taken off for Europe with some optimism, my usual zest for Zist (the retreat center) is numbed by the time I reach Penzberg, Germany. Normally I wake up before dawn, make coffee or strong ginseng tea, and read or write until Carl pokes his head in the door and we finish the pot and talk before it's time to teach. For ten years this has been the pattern. Now I don't wake up. Since he's teaching in the mornings, I make no effort to rouse myself. Carl knows I am struggling for my life, but he, too, thinks I will be healthy again. I wish he would tell me what to do, but he won't, of course. Damn it. I want an authority figure.

I don't write much either this time. Dutifully I do make some lists. It is what we ask patients to do, and I have been exhibiting classic denial.

What the Tumor Is Telling Me

- Change my life or die—I have a choice.
- It reminds me of how miserable I have been.

- I am in circumstances that are far too isolating.
- I was no longer curious.
- I was in a deep depression from which there just seemed to be no escape.
- There was no joy.
- My kids had exhausted my soul.
- Frank and I are no longer so deeply connected; we're bored, untrusting.
- I hated working as a paper-pusher for the journal.
- I could see no way out of anything except by death.
- I had extreme and unexpressed anger that had never been brought to the surface.
- My body had become a stew of things that I'd used in trying to make myself feel better, such as hormones and hormone precursors.
- This had been a year of profound loss—loss of the birds, of the kids, and of excitement.

Well, I'm getting pretty good at listing my woes.

I prepare a second list, which is supposed to consist of ideas on how to proceed. In retrospect, though, some of the items on this list seem to stray from the topic; many reflect what I have done rather than what I should do.

What to Do?

- Learned of the great love and support that surround me.
- Work with the dark and mysterious realms.
- Had some fun—especially with Judy in England.
- Slowed down my daily pace.
- Quit my position at the journal.
- Rethought living circumstances.
- Asked some people to stay away until I can regroup.
- Shifted slightly (at least in my own mind) my relationship with the kids. They are making their own choices, and I can accept them.
- Am a little more trusting in intuition and wisdom.
- Am moving forward on two books.

I do try to register my imagery in writing: starve the cells, take away their fuel, aim a p53 beam at them (p53 is the gene that causes cancerous cells to self-destruct), and give the suggestion that the retina will reattach. I imagine staying open to love and prayer while I do the mistletoe injections.

Carl keeps reminding me to pay attention to my "inner wisdom." My inner wisdom is telling me that I'm getting sick and tired of seeing no change in positive directions. So I decide to up the ante on the mistletoe and go for the highest strength. I arrange to have it delivered to Santa Fe by the time I get home.

The weather is bad, so we don't do the usual walking. The group is wonderful. I tell them a piece of my journey. It snows the last day—an early winter—and I take a picture of Carl and me. We look normal, or as normal as we ever do.

The Event

{November 11}

WHEN I GET HOME, the extra-strength mistletoe is waiting. Since I had been using Series I in Germany, I figure I'll just continue upping the dose, so instead of starting at the beginning of the series, I inject the most potent three vials over the following six days. Although everything that happened next could be attributed to the mistletoe, that wouldn't be fair. I'm changing my life here. I've been the target of thousands of prayers. I'm getting halfway serious about wanting to stay alive. I certainly intend to hang on until December so I can go to Kona Village in Hawaii on vacation, for one thing.

———◇———

Four days later I really feel good. Odd things are happening before my very eyes. I see cells and movements that look familiar. Some cells approach others, some disappear, and others develop blebs and go away. There are circular gold halos that move and surround cells. I can see this even with my eyes open. By now I have very limited vision, incidentally, but can still detect form and some color and movement. Fascinating. I've seen this stuff before. So I get out some immunology textbooks and a video we have on the immune system, photographed through a scanning electron microscope.

That's it: I'm watching my own immunology. This is not imagery, sports fans. I can see it, so it must be happening in front of my retina. I try to control some of the action, but I really can't tell the "good guys" from the "bad guys," so I just watch.

We have dinner with Barb and Larry Dossey, who ask about my imagery. I groan, because no one would believe what I am watching in my eye, but I tell them anyway. "But," I reiterate, "this is not imagery. I am seeing this for real." Larry volunteers that the retina, in a dark room, can register a single photon, which means that the eye is incredibly sensitive to the smallest particle of light or energy, and that I might well be viewing my own immune system at work.

I am higher than a kite. After dinner I am absolutely sure that remission is under way. I see blue. Can't remember the last time that happened. I leap around as I pack my suitcase.

I boarded the airplane for Washington, D.C., on November 16 to speak to the Music Therapy Conference and felt fabulous. I even bought a T-shirt and some earrings at the airport. Signs of life. You just don't feel in the mood for shopping when you're not sure you'll be around much longer. I didn't want anything new that was going to last longer than I would, and that included canned goods. As things turned out, though, it wasn't until at least six weeks later that I would remember my purchases and take the new things out of the bag.

In my journal I wrote, "Three more days, I believe, until an epiphany." (How would I have known that?) My traveling library consisted solely of a book by Saint John of the Cross about the Dark Night of the Soul, which was odd because I usually carry an extra bag just for books. The volume begins, "All dark nights are times of sheer grace." How perfect, I thought. The wisdom of a more contemplative life was being forced on me, and little did I know that I would get the hang of the Dark Night business through firsthand experience right downtown in our nation's capital city.

During the trip I continued to watch the mesmerizing display of immunology or whatever it was.

Either before falling asleep around midnight or maybe during a waking spell early the next morning, I scribbled notes on a yellow pad about something I had discovered the day before. It was about Frank. He and I had been turning outward, but not necessarily moving away from each other, long before the Grim Reaper diagnosis. Usually this was not obvious even to us because we treated each other with tenderness, publicly and privately, and had probably had only ten big, bad fights in almost a quarter of a century. But on this day I had found out that I no longer knew who he was, what he thought, or even where he went every day. We had seriously different windows on the social construction of reality as well as on right and wrong doing in human relationships. More than a failure of intimacy or interpersonal isolation, this bordered dangerously on sheer madness, and I felt I must try to do something about it. I stuffed the notepad into a suitcase and did not find it, or think about what I had written, for at least four months.

The morning of November 17, I woke up at 4:00 A.M., feeling as if acid had been poured into my eye, and looked over at the nightstand to see whether something might have been there that could have spilled. I rummaged through my luggage to find the sample of Ultram, a pain reliever that does not reduce inflammation. I had brought only two tablets and took them both. From this point on I instinctively avoided any anti-inflammatory agents because decreasing the inflammatory process did not feel correct. I was supposed to speak at 1:00 that afternoon and then leave at 3:00 to fly to California.

I asked for a wake-up call at 8:00, thinking I would get up and go find Mark Rider, a former student and now colleague, and listen to the beginning of the conference. Instead, I got some ice for my eye from the machine down the hall and put the cold plastic bag on my face for an hour or so. Then I got dressed in my "speaker suit," the beautiful yellow skirt and sweater from Austria, a charcoal silk jacket, and a hand-painted silk scarf.

The conference room was as cold as a meat locker. I went back to my room. Finally I got my luggage packed, dragged it downstairs, and returned to the conference room, which had gotten even colder.

My talk is the opener for the afternoon. It is on miraculous healing and is based on material Stan Krippner and I had just written for a book on anomalous phenomena, bravely published by the American Psychological Association. Sometimes I just can't stand the irony and paradox of my life in show biz. My topic is miracles, and I'm about to drop dead in public.

Never, in twenty-five years, have I had to leave a podium. Through all the kids' trauma, jet-lagged mornings, flu, pneumonia, sundry relationship crises, you name it, I got on stage and stayed there. From Japan to Germany to Argentina and back, I never missed a beat. People who speak publicly will understand: you usually get energized by a crowd, you rise to the occasion.

I stopped talking after thirty minutes and apologized. I could not even manage to sit at the end of a table designated for the panel. My body had entered into some foreign territory. It wasn't as if I were going to faint. I've fainted plenty since I was a baby. I'm a fainter, and they thought I had a heart condition. No, not fainting time. I rolled my luggage back to my room, thankful that I had not yet checked out, and fell into bed. Cold, cold fire.

Some weeks later a participant wrote to me about an altered-state experience she'd had during my lecture, in which the cold had transported her into another landscape. Cold drafts often accompany visits from the "afterlife," and maybe the folks in the afterlife were a-coming after me.

My eye and nose were gushing faucets of tears and mucus, and the left side of my face was swelling up and becoming unrecognizable even to me. It was distorted, like when you look into one of the crazy mirrors in a carnival fun house (if anybody alive still remembers those). I was immobilized by nausea. Every time I sat up or turned over, I threw up, and I had to crawl into the bathroom a couple of times. The silver thing they put over the plates for my breakfast room service became a vomit receptacle because eventually I could no longer manage to crawl to the bathroom. *Cold fire.* I was on cold fire.

I barely remember calling Mo, but I told her I wouldn't be there that night—I was so sick. Good-bye. The next day, and the day after, I realized I was still completely dressed and had my boots on—the happy outfit I had bought precisely a year ago that very week.

I finally got into my pajamas, put the yellow sweater back on, and switched to the other bed for a change of scenery. I guess by now I must have been moving around a little, at least to the toilet when vomiting ceased and diarrhea commenced. Barbara Rohrer, who had organized the conference, phoned a few times to suggest that I call the hotel doctors. Each time I promised her I would in a few hours. Calls came in from Mo and Judy. Frank phoned several times to remind me to order room service and eat something sweet. I did order room service once a day for the next four days. I probably cleaned out the minibar trying to stay hydrated and developed a fondness for nonalcoholic beer, which seemed to settle my stomach. The food was far better than in a hospital, and in one of my more lucid moments I was thinking, "Well, this isn't a bad way to go. Room service, housekeeping that is unobtrusive, and better than a hospital, for sure. I'm wearing a suitable outfit and have a religious book open on the bed." And I also think, "How ideal for me. I am alone, like the *Bone People* lady, and could do this nowhere else. If I were home, I would be tending to business no matter how bad I felt. There are always caves and cabins in the woods in which to do this sort of thing, but they don't have room service. No, this is just perfect. A fine hotel."

Andy Weil is there for some conference and finds out I'm under the weather, so to speak. He calls, and I tell him I have the flu, because that's all I can think of to call it. He gave me some suggestions to combat the nausea. He knows about the ocular melanoma, and I tell him that is where the flu is settling, but I am unable and embarrassed to tell him how bad I feel, and certainly nothing about the cold fire or the massive swelling going on my left eye. It looks as if the iris were going to separate from the sclera (the white part).

I call the house doc, and he orders some antibiotics, nose spray, and sugar syrup for an upset stomach. He asks whether I want him to come by my room, and I assure him that what he is prescribing will fix me up and I don't need a visit. I know that Jim Gordon, my colleague and traveling companion to the Balkans, is around the corner and would be there in a millisecond if called, but at this stage I need solitude and would not be good company. In retrospect it's clear that I am protecting myself from medicine, even of the alternative kind. Mark stops by, and I apologize for the way I look. Mark and I have not seen each other for about ten years, and I must look like an old witch—or perhaps more like Frankenstein's monster.

———◇———

Today, the nineteenth of November, is to be my day of epiphany, according to my own prognostications and maybe according to Steve

Wright's repeated visions of nineteen, the nineteen candles in the healing ceremony, the nineteen golden threads.

Wow. I can't get out of bed. Nothing is familiar; my body and mind are tilted. My eye is swelling up still more, but this is the least of my worries. Mostly I'm concerned about the cold fire. I call Good Doc, who is monitoring my situation as much as I'll allow, and he asks what color my eye is. I reply, "Red and blue." I ask him whether there is anything else I can do, and he figures it is conjunctivitis, combined with the flu, and will not affect the tumor.

I happen to have a prescription for Ambien, order a refill from the pharmacy, and am absolutely sure security thinks I am going to off myself with it. Reps from the security staff keep checking on me. Ambien is a sleep medication that clears in a hurry: you get about four hours of sleep, and then it's gone and the pain dragon rears its head again. I let housekeeping in to clean the bathroom only once that I remember. I keep scheduling and then postponing the trip home. (My eye is hurting and swelling up for the first time in weeks as I write this. Oh, God. Let's not do this again.)

Frank would have to go teach the final phase of our Year Long Training program in California alone because I couldn't get out of the bed in D.C. We have conducted these training sessions on imagery and mind-body consciousness four weekends a year at various locations for health-care professionals. They were the creative product of our mutual careers, the best of our work, and we have done them together for ten years. This phase of the training focused on ritual and community support. The group did several healing rituals for me. Later some of the participants told me that Frank had been pensive and noncommittal, and when they tried to comfort him, he assured them that everything was going to be just fine and it was only the flu.

The hotel agreed to let me stay a few more days but doubled the rate. Who cares? I couldn't move. I argued a little and then hung up.

My spiritual tools were so thin. I listened to the shamanic drumming tape a few times, and then either it or the machine failed. I set it aside and did not find it again, like my airport purchases, until many weeks later when I unpacked my suitcase. I tried to imagine myself being held by two white angels. They seemed to be male and strong, if slightly contrived. I surrendered. This, I find later, *is* the Dark Night—when you are totally naked and bowed low, when your spiritual allies have deserted you. No mantras, no prayers, no voices from angels or saints or dead relatives. You are not in the void, you *are* the void—and hanging on to the sides of the bed for dear life. Funny, I always thought the Dark Night was something like depression. I know depression. This is different.

As I learned more afterward, I came to realize that I was probably in shock from an immune hyperstimulation. Mistletoe liberates or stimulates tumor necrosis factor (TNF). TNF is normally created by certain immune cells, and it is also stimulated by the proliferation of white blood cells, such as T-cells, that kill cancer. But excessive amounts of TNF are associated with septic and toxic shock.

Mistletoe also stimulates the interleukins, proteins that activate the immune system. I was also pumped up on Cellular Forté, which stimulates natural killer cell activity. I can recite a litany of chemicals in which I was awash. But at the time I and everyone else thought I had that demon flu that was going around, and of course, we simply do not know.

Mo called and told me to try to get home, get a wheelchair ordered at the airport, make sure I get on first class.

"Mo, you don't understand. I need litter bearers." I am always thrilled when I can inject a little humor into the dying process. "Oh, better stay there, then," she said, in her deep, no-bullshit voice.

———◇———

Finally, on November 21, I dragged myself out of bed and flew home after five days in the hotel of doom. The conference paid my entire bill. I protested feebly as I staggered out, but Barbara Rohrer said, "Just say thank-you. Don't argue." I sent my honorarium check back uncashed.

After a layover in Denver, I managed to get to the Albuquerque airport, but not home. I guess I was feverish, but strangely so. Still that cold inner fire—as if neither it nor I would register on a thermometer. Frank was flying in that night also, so I left a message for him at the airport to be broadcast by the PA system when he arrived, then trudged over to the Wyndham Hotel dragging my big bags. Looking back, I don't know how I navigated that far or how Frank ever found me, given the dubious reliability of airport PA systems, but we'd always had radar for each other, even in Home Depot.

———◇———

Frank drove me home the next day, turned down the covers, and I crawled into our big bed, with its vistas of distant mountains and extinct volcanoes. When I managed to get a look at my left eye, it was frightening. The eye had doubled in size, and where the sclera joins the iris, it looked more and more as if it was going to split. All the pain, which had previously been diffuse, settled behind the eye and felt just like a boil localizing before it erupts.

Now I was just starting to entertain faint suspicions that this might not exactly be the flu, but it wasn't until Carl called (a few days later, maybe?) and said, "Not in my personal experience, nor in my clinical experience, have I ever seen the flu in one eye. People don't get the flu in one eye. And you don't have the symptoms of conjunctivitis either." He seemed excited.

I still held on to the sides of the bed. Behind me I had several vials of holy water that had been sent from around the world, and I was anointing my eye whenever I could. Figure it's best to cover your bases. Another landscape appeared. Angles and lines. Black-and-white line forms. I tried to make out figures but couldn't. If anything, the figures looked like mechanical toys, and it was probably the disruption of rods and cones (rods and cones are the tiny receptors in the retina that pick up black and white or color, respectively). If you can imagine a thick fluid flung at a window and drops running down the window pane, that is what I saw. There were spots of color flowing through periodically. Then I saw what looked like the earth during a quake, rippling movement, and crevices. This I actually saw, but I also had an image of a blue door, which appeared momentarily and then disappeared. Since I don't have many visual images, it startled me.

I'm trying to report all this because I think this is what happens when every immune component fires off at once and heads for your eye. If anyone else goes through this, he or she would need more help than I was able or willing to request. The pain was formidable, and although injections or suppositories would have taken the edge off, it didn't occur to me to take them. All I knew is that oral pain medications would not stay down, and I was afraid of getting slapped in the hospital if I complained too much. The usual method for treating eye inflammation is with cortisone, which, of course, inhibits the healing process. I wanted to give my eye a chance, even if it was a last-ditch effort.

I may or may not have blasted out my eye. But if any vision does return, it will be more than I would have had with radiation or eye removal, and the treatment I am experimenting with may prove to be more viable in preventing metastasis. Or it may simply prove to be crazy. Had I been able to reach Carl sooner, I might have gone through the process with more assurance—although I was too sick to be very scared. He called an anthroposophic doctor, who told him that what had happened was exactly what one would expect, or at least hope for, and that it was considered a special gift from God when the tumor is so directly targeted.

Thanksgiving and Transcendence

{November 23}

THIS MORNING I BOLTED UPRIGHT, amazed, and said, "I'm happy. My God, I feel happy." Something—it felt like God's breath—blew away the darkness that had held me captive for longer than I care to remember. Effortlessly, I was just filled with joy. I had awakened in a new body, to a new world, a place I scarcely remembered. For at least the past six years, nothing could drive a wedge into the hovering sorrow, the heaviness, and the sense of loss of purpose. Nothing stopped the ebbing stream of my vitality or made the Life Force, the source of my vitality, come back—nothing in my yearning. No invitation was sufficient. My spiritual path had become weedy and was no longer negotiable. I was stripped, surrendering, and nearly unconscious.

This return of the Life Force was not of my doing. It was Grace. The Curse of Darkness was broken. The Eye became totally inconsequential. I was now larger than the Thing and never again went into the Valley of Fear of Medicine and Death. I had no time; I had to get on with living. Something *big* had happened, and whether it meant I was coming or going did not matter so much anymore. Energy for renegotiating life, however long that might be, surged through my veins. I was still very sick and could hardly walk, and the Thing was localizing even more, but that was all right, and I dozed, drifting in and out, for the rest of the day.

Mara Jan finally reached me by telephone. She had been trying to find me since November 17 because she was worried about what was happening. Like all the girlfriends, Mara Jan is abundantly endowed with intuition. She had also tracked my horoscope, and some celestial alarm bells were ringing.

"Who is taking care of you?" which is a Mara Jan–type question.

"Frank is in town."

"Anybody else?

"Barbie and Larry check in a couple of times a day. I keep asking them to assure me that I'm not crazy for using holy water instead of running to the hospital. I know they are worried because I'm babbling and only half conscious from the pain, and they would probably be more comfortable if I got some medical care. But I just can't. Larry keeps saying, 'You're in uncharted territory here,' but he's supportive, and this is not my first venture into strange seas." Mara Jan seemed pleased that locals were available to me, since the other girlfriends were so far away.

I kept a new journal right by my bed, hoping for action similar to yesterday's. This time I planned to record it. I tried to imagine the cancer cells, but they never felt quite real; my mind just never found them. All that I could see was a cup with liquid spewing, spilling out. I drew it and shrugged. It made no sense in my partial state of consciousness. After the fact it made all the sense in the world. The Thing had exploded, there were hemorrhages, vessels expanded hugely to accommodate the process, and the contents of the Thing were thrown at the anterior chamber of my eye.

Since the Event I've read much more about the healing process, which is strangely ignored and misunderstood. What happened to me is what happens. The body tries to fight an invader with a local reaction. Histamine is released (the tears), vessels expand so immune components can travel, the response is diffuse and then localizes. If this doesn't work, the whole body gets in gear: fever signals the systemic reaction. Why it could not have been gentler—a gradual cell death or apoptosis (the normal, preprogrammed cellular death), washing away the dead cells through the usual ways the eye drains—why it was so sudden, I didn't know, nor was there any explanation for how the Thing got so big in the first place or why it grew so fast. It does not seem appropriate for the eye to have had such a dramatic Event. The space is too small, the mechanisms too complicated. This must have been a desperate effort to expel what did not belong there.

———◇———

I received a healing E-mail from a San Francisco psychologist who was in our year-long training program held at the Dominican retreat at Santa Sabina, in San Rafael, California:

> Jeanne,
> You were deeply missed at Santa Sabina, and I hope that our prayers not only ended your flu but increased your healing abilities in general. Some priestess friends and I gathered for a full moon in Gemini / Sun in Sagittarius ritual last night. We called on Athena and Owl Spirit and journeyed with Owl to see, through Owl's eyes, the answers to our questions. This is a time to balance and rise above to find our paths. We each chose a feather from my air altar and used it for our journey, taking it with us. Others and I gathered the feathers on hikes and backpacking trips. My concern for you was one of the thoughts before I began the journey, and in today's meditation I got that maybe Owl would be helpful to you in your healing and quest to find a new vision of yourself. So an eight-day candle burns for you with a feather from my altar next to it and a prayer for Owl to guide you if you so choose. I will send the feather to you at the candle's end. Much love.

———◇———

Thanksgiving. Emily Hilburn Sell, my editor at Shambhala Publications and now my good friend, calls, and we talk for about two hours. I have agreed to revise *Imagery in Healing,* which is still widely used and quoted, but the research citations are shamefully out of date. Not until this very day would the thought of any revision or any new writing have been entertained. I was just too weary of work and life to give a good damn. Emily's timing is superb. My own mythic journey, the shifts forced on me away from biology to story and spirituality, a new sensitivity for both the value and the difficulty of imagery as a healing tool, and on and on. "You have your finger in the socket, so to speak. You need to write this now because nobody else can," she says. Emily and I discuss the amazing synchronicities between us, including the fact that we are both surviving on a drink made of raspberries and soy powder.

Most of the day Frank and I watch cowboy movies on TV. My eye hurt (no, *hurt* isn't the word, but I can't come up with a better one), so I just cuddle by him and listen. I do watch the very ancient *Son of Paleface* and laugh until I cry when Trigger gets in bed with Bob Hope. I fell in love with Roy Rogers when I saw him in his skivvies in that movie when I was about ten, so it was a historic occasion.

Frank and I have our traditional quiet dinner with Larry and Barbie Dossey and count our blessings—our enduring couples' relationship being a major one. Barbie is so very helpful on understanding eye pain: she's been there with her own corneal implant. Larry has found an article on hypnosis describing a woman who knew each part of her body intimately and could describe her eye, layer by layer. After dinner, a mighty fine one at the Inn of Anasazi, we take a stroll around the festive plaza, and the cold air hits my eye like a knife.

———◇———

The *Alternative Therapies* journal editors and my friend Bonnie, our publisher, gathered in Santa Fe a few days later. It was my first meeting after my hiatus and sabbatical. I hurt, but not so much. If I hadn't felt and looked a little better each day, I would have had my eye removed, no question. The pain had been almost unendurable, and if it had lasted any longer, it would not have been worth stubbornly hanging on even to anything as personal as a body part. I endured the meetings; tried to concentrate; drove, squinting into the setting sun; and did regular things. At night I fell gratefully into bed with an eye pillow over my eyes, at Barbie's suggestion. (The eye pillow, a lavender-filled silk rectangle, put slight pressure on my eyes and shut out the light.)

Meeting our new editor, William Faire, was one of the high points of this gathering, and he came into my life at just the right time to reinforce my independent path. Bill was a urologist at Memorial Sloan-Kettering Cancer Center. He is also chic, witty, and very wise. When Bill was diagnosed with colon cancer some years ago, his radical story made *The New Yorker*. Bill faced a sentence of death and defied it through his own devices. He researched herbs and mushrooms and other supplements and fed them to mice with tumors. Those that were taking the concoctions lived and the other mice died, so he took his own prescription.

———◇———

A message from Steve Wright arrived: "I wondered if something was up, as you had been in my mind intensely day after day. Sat with it, prayed, meditated, asking . . . what more should I do? Sudden reflection . . . have had two nights of short dreams with you and a swan . . . yes . . . and yesterday I went into Keswick, and there is a life-size swan (plastic!!!) in a display in a shop window. Perhaps I am missing something. I do not know. Do you have swans where you live???"

I wrote back that I didn't know about swans, but other people, including Carl, had seen swans or white birds around my invisible space. I like this image. White birds are angels to me, like my beloved cockatoo, J.C., and the two barely there guys that I had tried to entice into the hotel room of doom just the week before.

———◇———

Bonnie came to see me, and we sat on the pink-tinged rock formation, shot with streaks of quartz, behind my house drinking in at least a hundred miles of view. We stirred up the project cauldron together, and it was like the good old days. I had needed to leave the journal, for my own sake as well as for the growth of the publication. She asked, "Would you ever have resigned if we hadn't had a fight?" No, of course not. I would have continued to sit reading and writing, critiquing and bitching, day after day, out of loyalty to her, Larry, and whatever else was tied up into this package.

Today was also the beginning of the snot cascade, and faithful to my task as girl medical reporter, I have to record even these fairly disgusting events. Whatever was happening inside my eye, my sinuses were trying to wash it away. It is the oddest-tasting snot—never had anything like it. Not bad, just odd. Metallic. Clear, like cervical mucus when you ovulate. Or when the gag reflex is triggered. And profuse, especially in the mornings. It is coming from the sinus over and under the right part of my left eye—where the Thing was located. Nowhere else. Since summer, whenever I've touched the upper right part of my eye, over that sinus, it has drained. The MRI showed it to be full of something. As with the infected tooth directly below this area, no one who looked at me or my records saw any relationship between this and the Thing. What the hell do I know? Maybe they're right. No, they're not—and there I go talking to myself again.

I've probably lost all vision in the left eye, but I don't check. Am still too overwhelmed with the pain, the redness, and the swelling. My iris, normally green, is black. The white part is red. Aside from that, everything is OK.

On the last day of November, I prepare the following "update," which circulates via E-mail to several thousand people. Crystal Hawk and others send it to their respective circles. I send it with cards to Jim Lake, Larry LeShan, Margaret Christensen, and many others.

Dear Ones,

Thank you for being present with me during this difficult time of sheer grace and for your inquiries about my health and life. As I think most of you know, I came back last summer from working in the refugee camps, greatly touched, and prayed for a larger vision and new direction for my life. Be careful what you pray for. Within weeks I had a detached retina, lost vision (at least with my eye), and was diagnosed with an ocular melanoma. It had probably been with me for years. Such tumors grow slowly, and if they metastasize, it can be up to thirty years after the diagnosis. They are quite rare, as tumors go. The conventional treatments for a tumor this size are not exactly benign: eye removal or a big dose of radiation that would compromise the eye itself. Neither treatment would improve vision, obviously, nor provide any guarantee regarding quality or quantity of life, nor improve my sense of humor.

I've chosen another path for now. The tumor is highly immunoreactive, so I have sought therapies that stimulate the immune system. This makes sense to me, and you know how I feel about needing to find treatments that mesh with belief. Ideally my body will marshal its defenses and at least reduce the size of the tumor so that a lesser dose of radiation will be required or preferably make it go away altogether. The "biological alternatives" (now being called biological response modifiers, among other things) that I am using are not benign either but are reasonably well researched and are a standard part of medicine in much of Europe. They are doing what they are supposed to do, and I have only just now responded systemically (flu and fever) and with a tremendous local reaction, and so am dragging along, feeling like a case of one-eyed bubonic plague.

Now here's the real story. I am awed, humbled, and grateful beyond any words. The true medicines are the prayers, ceremonies, calls, E-mails, letters, songs, dreams, and gifts of your intentions and time and energy. Such caring is beyond anything I could have imagined, nothing that I know how to repay, and I can respond only with tears of gratitude. I feel surrounded by love and am certainly the most fortunate creature on earth. The healings have occurred at every layer of my being. My restless soul has been nurtured in profound ways. Humanity has reaffirmed itself. There are still healers in medicine and mystics and sages and wise men and women in abundance. I called on so many people, and everyone responded with great generosity of spirit.

I do not know what will happen to my physical eye—but I am fully ready for this dis-ease to pass. A great learning for me is that serious healing requires serious attention and that each act must be done with more awareness. Life needs to become a meditation (have read that somewhere). I initially tried to tack healing on to everything else in my busy life. It just doesn't work that way. So I am moving around more deliberately, choosing my activities with more consciousness.

I have not canceled any of my engagements for spring but will not add others for a year or so. Work is life, for me, and somehow that needs to be held in perspective. We are acting on some dreams that went by the wayside when we moved—gathering more of our beloved animals around us (all our animals died this year), finding a helper/caretaker, restructuring this huge property so we can offer sanctuaries to friends and families who need the healing space of a crystal mountain, and living more in community.

So many ask me what you can do. You can just be there in thoughts with me. On days when the stark terror creeps in, it helps if I know people are absolutely trusting in the outcome. I need to hear your stories and experiences, the strengths you found when you were on the edge. I need your humor and laughter. I just need people in my life right now to support my nontraditional way of doing things.

Frank is well. We're taking care of each other as best we can, and maybe that's just what old sweethearts do.

I love you all so much.

Jeanne

The response is loving and tremendous.

Saint Lucy's Days

{December 2}

DAVID LUKOFF SHARED my letter with the Saybrook faculty. They did a healing ceremony for me on December 2—the day of Saint Lucy, patron of vision. "Thanks," he said in a card that accompanied a beautiful crystal that had been the centerpiece for the ritual, "for helping us flex our transpersonal muscles." It was, of course, my privilege. The Saybrook faculty astounded me. I just had no idea about the depths of their caring. In October they had obtained a medal of Saint Lucy and passed it around to each member of the faculty, who blessed it with his or her intentions for me. The thought of having this faculty, in all its contentious glory, spend time and energy rallying around my healing has been one of the most touching events in this time outside of time. I have never taken Saint Lucy off, except once to have a massage. In the usual postmassage state of trance, I left her and panicked, only to discover that within minutes she had found her way back to me.

Frank would be leaving for Indiana to do our training alone once again. It didn't take me terribly long to decide not to go. I don't care what "they" say, riding in an airplane is a bit of a physical challenge even for people in the best of health, so it couldn't be good for someone with a problematic eye.

We spent the night near the airport so Frank could leave very early. When he left, I asked him to cover me with as many blankets as he could find. This was the very last day of the cold fire. I was finally able to get up, navigate home, buy poinsettias, and do some Christmas decorating.

I have a telephone appointment with Mark Rennecker, my medical detective. He's been poking around, has letters from eye docs, and has done some research. Right from my first conversation with Mark, I was impressed with his medical knowledge about ocular melanoma. If he knows this much about other conditions, he's a genius. He is not entirely convinced I've been properly diagnosed and thinks that, if I have, I've been overdiagnosed. He finds too many discrepancies in my "case." The bleeds and so on should not have been ignored. We talk for about an hour. He is very curious about my eye explosion, the snot cascade, what "alternatives" I am using. I tell Mark I would only be interested in a vaccine treatment at this point. He's going to continue the research, and we'll talk after Christmas.

———◇———

I receive a fax from Christian Buettner, the German physician I have never met who is advising Carl and me on the mistletoe. He says, "Dear Jeanne, after the phone call I felt for sure that you will find your very personal way of working with your cancer." With the fax comes a beautiful drawing of a mistletoe plant.

———◇———

I canceled more medical appointments that had been assigned to me by fax. Same old song and dance. I wouldn't have been able to get affordable airline tickets at that late date, and my eye was too sore for a sonogram anyway. I knew that with all the inflammation, the pressure to get rid of the eye or use steroids to reduce the swelling would be increased, and there was simply no point in making any more perturbations either in me or in the system about me at that time. I needed a break from medical treatment and decided to extend it until I reached a place where I didn't make the doctors so nervous, they didn't make me so nervous, and/or I didn't give a good shit what they did to me. So it was either establish trust or succumb, and in the meantime I was going to pretend I had a life. I also needed a rest from just everything, including all the pills and potions.

We left for Kona Village on the Big Island of Hawaii on December 11, to play and be with Mo, Judy, and their families for the week. It was supposed to be a healing time for me, and it was very hard to admit I was sick, but I was. About every three days I had an "eye attack," for no obvious reason. Reading was impossible, so I mostly stared inward or gazed outward to the ocean surrounding this Healing Island, crocheted, and visited, but not often. I clearly wasn't very good company, but Frank was also subdued, and we stayed quiet and alone.

Body work every day. And a sauna. And a workout. We figured we walked at least five miles just to get to meals each day. This does not exactly sound like being on a sickbed. There are two main categories of people: those who are sick but act well and those who are really well (or well enough) but pretend they are sick.

We were presented with a huge outdoor buffet for lunch each day, and dinner was a feast for the senses. I only ate meat for lunch and dinner, and hash browns and raspberries for breakfast, to everyone's disgust.

A little interjection here about diet. I am a former right-wing diet fanatic. We did the "Ornish diet" when Frank had a heart attack. I learned how to cook again, and my assistant, Beverly Messenger, and I shopped, chopped, and moved into the kitchen for the better part of each day. I humbly apologize to anyone who has ever been offended by my fanaticism. Under stress I can't eat. When I don't eat, I feel bad. My body craved protein—contrary to most of the advice of the cancer diet folks—and that is all that would go down for months.

One day in Hawaii I peer into my eye and observe that the iris is still mostly black. Shocking. But some white is to be seen amid the red.

Time to go home, darn it.

And time to get ready for Christmas. I got some decorations at the hobby shop on December 22—so late, in fact, that they asked me whether I was buying for next year.

I guess I am still sick. I stay in bed until ten or so and then take a nap. While out shopping today, I look in the car mirror and *eeks*. In the sunlight my pupil appears to be covered with a glob of yellow debris, which has probably been there since the Event but just went unnoticed because of the black and the red. There are at least three chunks of something in it. I also see blood under my iris and in the circle surrounding the pupil. There are streaks of black in my iris. No wonder

I can't see. But there is a little green on the top edge. This becomes my biofeedback for the coming weeks—watching the amount of green increase.

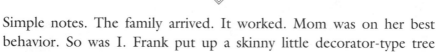

Simple notes. The family arrived. It worked. Mom was on her best behavior. So was I. Frank put up a skinny little decorator-type tree before they came. We had a lovely Christmas. My brother Gary did the emotional balancing act for the family, as usual.

Jim Lake wrote to me on this Christmas Eve. I had shared my experience with his candle on the strange Vision Quest night on the dark mountain and asked for his feedback. He gave me a deep well of symbolism, and it concerns my learning a way of seeing that is necessary to guide me from an unknown place of darkness to light and to home, which is always within. "In showing the world (including me) that a teacher like yourself can trust that the light is inside, that real seeing does not require eyes, you provide me with a liberating understanding of my own parallel journey that is sometimes synchronistic with yours and all who strive to see clearly in a world where there is often loss, often obscuring, dangerous fog—even in high places where one can expect to find great insight."

Jim and I continue to weave around each other. He treated my son for a time when he was in the psychiatric unit, so he is connected to me in the most intimate way—through my beloved Chase. I'm certain, too, that my disturbed, sensitive son shared his view of my maternal failings with Jim.

On this evening I received a fax from Christian Buettner: "Merry Christmas, dear Jeanne, and a good and happy New Year!" He included a poem from Rudolf Steiner with the promise, "The light of the sun brightens all space when dark night is past."

Young Things

{December 26}

MY FOLKS LEFT, and Brianne, my twelve-year-old granddaughter, came for the week. She is the joy of my life. She has always been sensitive and knew when she was only months old how to interact with all the personalities of her multiple grandparents. But this year she was even more solicitous than usual, taking care of me when she could and carefully gauging my energy levels so she could adjust hers to match.

We went to town every day, ate fast food, and shopped. I tried to appear well but took a nap in the afternoons while Brianne read one of her many books. She went with me to Roland, who does my hair, and I watched her concerned little face, as she watched me, when I told him I would need to have my bangs on the left side slightly cover my eye. I guessed then that she had been told I was very ill, so after we left the salon, I told her about my eye but said that I thought it was getting well. Being around an allegedly half-dead Grandma Jeanne must have been a burden on her young mind, and I wanted to relieve her.

She reads all the time and has an amazing ability to express herself verbally. She is truly the grandchild of my heart, if not my blood, and when I am with her, time stands still.

———◇———

Later in the week we get the puppies. They are another "what are the odds?" story. On the way back from Kona, we stopped to change planes in Denver. I bought a paper to check the classifieds. A litter of puppies (Samoyeds) is listed in the 505 area code. I think, "It must be a misprint," because 505 is New Mexico. No mistake. They were in Taos, but the litter that was advertised had been sold. Another one will be ready in mid-January. Then yesterday the breeder called and said, "I have very good news for you. Two puppies are still available, a male and a female." We know they are ours. Big honkin' doggies—they were born October 2 and now weigh about twenty-five pounds each. Spirit and Angel. The house is filled with puppy energy and puppy smells. We settle on crate training—and buy a big one that's parked by our bed. All they want is love, and so do we. Match made in heaven.

Brianne and I carry the doggies around, staggering under their weight, and try to puppy-proof a few rooms. Angel's full name is really Angelina Hernandez Fernandez Gonzalez Lopez. Her ears perk up to the music of her name, and she is the bigger and bossier and wants more kisses. Spirit Dawg seems more thoughtful and wise. I love them so much, I want to pinch and pet and squeeze them all the time.

A missive came from Etzel Cardena, an anthropologist, friend, writer, and editor:

> Hi, Jeanne:
> I just recently came back from a trip to Spain and Portugal. In Raga, Portugal, I saw a sculpture of the Saint of Vision, and I asked her to assist you every way possible. Will you let me know how you are doing these days? Healing and soothing wishes for the year 2000.

Life Returns

{January 1}

NEW YEAR'S EVE with the Dosseys; we eat dinner at one of the best restaurants, as usual, and share prayers of gratitude. Afterward Frank and I do our usual retrospective and prospective look at life. He asks what is going to happen to me. I tell him I don't know. How would I know? Everything has been a big surprise this past year.

But on this day, along with the turning of the century, there is a second turnaround. My energy has started to come back. I'm restless. Slowly, molecule by molecule, there is some change in the eye, change that would be detectable only by its owner.

By January 6 I knew for sure I was getting well. There are several things you don't do if you think your days are numbered (besides not buying items that will outlast you): you don't have your furniture reupholstered, get your teeth cleaned, or learn new software programs. With some pride, after four hours of effort, I mastered PowerPoint so I could make my own slides. My furniture doesn't need reupholstering, so I guess I'll start thinking about a trip to the dentist next.

A dream came in from Steve:

> You are in a strange, windy place, like a wind tunnel, passageway canyon of some sort. You are moving very fast, your hair streams

179

out behind, yet your feet don't seem to move. There are people lining the passageway, yet they turn from you as if in fear, afraid to look you in the eye, for your right eye has changed from a dark, shadowy place to a brilliant point of light, surrounded by two small but distinct concentric circles. It is this eye that now people fear, for with it you see right through them, see them as they really are, and to some this is very frightening. So they cast their gaze away from you, afraid to be seen by this eye, as you move fast and past them.

As before, I do not understand this; I simply report what I see.

———◇———

Mark Rennecker and I had another consultation in mid-January. He sent me the product of his investigations before Christmas, but I hid the thick binder from myself for about two weeks. I did not want to face the medical realities over the holidays. He told me in his letter to use the information for my imagery and information and not be derailed by the morbidity and mortality figures. I know this. These are my lines. I just forgot to use them on myself. When I finally did open the package, I was more curious than upset. The letters about me were vague, did not describe any detail that was useful, and were primarily a recitation of our conversations during office visits. The articles were quite helpful. One was from the John Wayne Cancer Institute, where a "vaccine" program is being conducted for patients with cutaneous melanoma. I called to find out whether the program accepts patients with ocular melanoma. The person who answered the phone yelled the question to somebody across the room. The answer yelled back was "No."

From the articles in Mark's package, I also learned the difference between immunotherapy and chemotherapy. Basically it is one of speed. Immunotherapy works slowly but more effectively. So when I spoke with Mark, I had an agenda. First, I wanted to express how appalled I was at the treatment for this problem and at the failure to move ahead with clinical trials on immunotherapy or vaccines. He said, "I think if you were to look closely at most cancer treatment, you would feel the same way." Of course, and I do. And I always was horrified, but especially, though, by the lackadaisical attitude about removing an eye. My eye.

One of the articles Mark sent described controlled trials in which patients were randomly assigned to eye removal or the radioactive plaque procedure. After the study was over, the comment was made that many of those who had had an eye removed could well have bene-fited from the plaque instead, which often partly spares vision. I wonder how that made those people feel who had lost an eye due to the ran-domness of their assignment. Or did they care? And I wonder how long the study went on before the researchers figured this out.

My second point was that I wanted to tell Mark about my continued progress and plan. At this date I had no intentions of submitting myself for standard treatment, nor did I wish to have a sonogram, for the reasons I've mentioned before—including discomfort, the test's lack of precision, and the anxiety it would create in the eye docs and me. Mark was still in agreement: he'd do the same. The unusual events preceding the time of diagnosis, the bleeds, and so on, and my remarkable re-sponse to the mistletoe (or whatever) should be taken into consider-ation, he said. I told him I still would only consider a vaccine at this point. It has great potential, being the most logical treatment.

We agreed that I would try to contact a hospital in the Netherlands where a study may be under way or at least treatment may be available. Mark suggested that I call and "chat" with them, to get information that may be off the record. I didn't mind doing that, since I could speak their scientific lingo, but what they eventually told me amounted to the same razzmatazz: go get your eye removed or burned out, and they recommended the same circuitous route, the same eye docs. After that I had to talk to myself again, about how immunoreactive the Thing is, whether it really is melanoma and not some other anomalous phenome-non like a bleed, and how many "spontaneous remissions" have been reported.

Mark asked me whether I had a timeline. I replied, "No," and told him what I'd learned about the slow nature of immune therapy. He agreed—but only because of the very strange nature of my "case." I, too, usually suggest that patients establish some time frame for how long they are willing to undergo treatment (or any other approach) before they reconsider their direction.

Mark read several alternative diagnoses to me, but they didn't seem to fit, except for "uveal bleed." He said, "But it just seems to be a default diagnosis, what they call something that doesn't fit any other category."

Mark has gotten me to thinking, which may be a good or bad sign. If I had gone to specialists over the last few months, I would now be minus a uterus, a few teeth, an eye, and eventually a lot of other facial tissue from radiation. In addition I would have had surgery on a sinus, which would have meant a total of at least four general anesthesias and quite a few "conscious sedations." It would be difficult enough to predict the normal course of recovery from so many chemicals and violations, but my peculiar and negative reaction to drugs—and especially anything sedating—would have exponentially increased the chances of treatment-related side effects. Several ultrasensitive and aware women I know who are also physicians have been monitoring their own recovery from chemicals and surgery, and their estimates far exceeded anything I would have predicted based on my own experience. Truth be told, it may take more than a year to be detoxified following general anesthesia.

Well, anyway, there's no telling what else is wrong with me and what might need to be removed or inserted if I were to be carefully inspected, as many insisted should be done. God save me from careful inspection. God save us all from careful inspection. I figure that, as things now stand, I'm still doing the work of ten good men, looking at least ten years younger than my age (although I would prefer fifteen), and life has some luster, albeit muted.

———◇———

Frank and I began Phase I of our year-long training at the most idyllic of all settings, the Dominican retreat at Santa Sabina, in San Rafael, California. My spiritual greed overcame me: should I go to the gardens, the chapels, or the new straw-bale hermitage? The setting facilitates the teaching and healing process for professionals who are often "wounded healers" themselves.

Working with Frank was a pleasure this go-round, and I learned from him because he had new material from working with the cancer patients and the Indians at Eight Northern Pueblos. I was very happy to be "back on the road again." I had missed the teaching and even the airports. Whenever possible, though, I ducked into my room and put on my eye pillow.

January 23 was the day I sat down to outline my experiences over the past year, in hopes of eventually ending up with a book. When Barbie and Larry Dossey inquired about my treatment last week, I gave a brief description of the mistletoe but not the kill-or-cure routine, because most people really don't want to hear the whole business. Even Frank does not know what I've been doing. But wait, maybe this is medical history. (It is for me, anyway, regardless of the outcome.) So I wrote a brief summary for the Dosseys and just kept on writing. Turns out, I wasn't sure just what did or didn't constitute the treatment, any more than I knew what the dis-ease was really called.

This did not feel like a particularly good day to begin. Maybe my reluctance was an anniversary reaction. It was exactly six months ago today that Eye Man in the Big City gave me the Grim Reaper news. Last night was bad, and I have given up on ever seeing out of the eye again. Progress is so slow. And today I'd just wanted to sleep until it (whatever "it" is) is over.

Mistletoe day. I have gone down to the weakest series of the preparations. After the November Fireball in the Eye Event, it seemed that what I needed was a maintenance dose and not the killer-diller one. The Thing itself appears to be gone, I am in repair mode, and I just want the mistletoe to remind my immune system to stay on patrol. I also take a slug of supplements. Yesterday I worked out at the spa like a son of a b, took two saunas, and stayed moving most of the day. Am poised to begin a kamikaze routine again if I don't see some change. My eye socket is sore, and something drains when I rub under the outside of the eye, where I imagine a drain would be. Light comes in, but it's like looking through a three-inch-thick black cracked glass—no shape, no form, some afterimages when I look at the sun. Enough light enters from the not-so good eye to block the afterimages unless I cover that eye. Light is not image.

By a couple of days later, things had improved a bit. Went out with the Dosseys last night. They can usually take my mind off anything, but still, I couldn't wait to get home to bed. The pain was now completely gone. The area of yellow debris that had covered my pupil since my eye exploded in November was getting smaller and thinner, but oh so slowly, molecule by molecule, and light was coming in only photon by photon.

Had an E-mail from Steve Wright in England, who had dreamed that I was just fine. Thanks, Steverino.

———◇———

The next day, though, I was feeling really weird. (Enzymes? Coffee?) Last night I had a glass of red wine and realized it was going straight to my eye, so who knows? For the first time I dreamed that a little vision had returned. The night before I woke around 4:00 a.m. from some sort of dream, but it was more like a body sensation. Someplace in my head or neck, something was struggling to readjust or get back in line. Like millions of moving parts. Wish I could recapture this. It didn't feel negative at all.

I am feeling pissy again, irritated with small things, and the same old concerns have started to recycle like garbage. I must be getting well or needing exercise.

God, I'm sick of all this, and I've only been at it a few months. People with diabetes and arthritis and other chronic problems who, after years of self-care, finally just throw up their hands, turn their faces to the wall, and quit taking care of themselves have a point. Who wants to live like this?

I'm still working, back as journal editor, at Saybrook, and on the road teaching and giving lectures about whatever is on my mind— usually health, imagery, and the healing nature of relationships.

This massive change, and yet the same old sixes and sevens, reminds me of a favorite poem:

> My boat has struck something deep.
> Sounds, waves, silence.

Maybe nothing has happened, or maybe I'm in the middle of my new life.

Meditation Medicine

{January 29}

A PSYCHIATRIST FRIEND suggested that Frank and I do a "medicine" session to see whether we could move out of a stuck place. We agreed it would be timely but not especially wise. The medicine she suggested was MDMA, or Ecstasy, a street drug formerly (and now secretly, but frequently) used in therapy. Frank and I have been consulting with a group of researchers who have actually had FDA approval to do initial testing on the chemical, and the next step is to administer it to cancer patients who are statistically unlikely to live more than a couple of months. The chemical has a well-deserved reputation for allowing people to open their hearts and gain perspective on their own stories. It is not the "fast horse" of LSD or some plant medicines, such as ayuaska, but is fairly gentle and predicable. MDMA also relieves pain for a substantial length of time, a fact not well known even to aficionados.

I got very excited about the research because, for about two hours during the altered state caused by the chemical, there is the possibility of classically conditioning a response to relieve pain by using imagery. In other words, if a person listens to an imagery tape during the MDMA peak period, the imagery tape, used at any time after the session, may be a source of pain control.

We decided to try to replicate the altered state created by MDMA as we remembered it, but without the chemical. It would not be good either for my metabolism or for Frank's professional reputation, because of his work on the Indian pueblos with drug and alcohol addiction. But I was also aware that Frank had allocated just so much of his time to me and us, and the rest must be reserved for his needs. In what bucket was this day going to be dropped? Our intentions were set to focus primarily on opening up a new chapter in my life, so it would likely be debited from my twelve-week account. No longer sick Saint Jeanne, I was starting to remember some things I had tried to forget, like the time deal.

We got out "traveling music," candles, incense, held each other, breathed together, and tried to focus on the bond between us. My eye seemed unimportant, and neither of us thought or spoke of it. The message from our meditations was that there was nothing much more I should or could do. But the next day I had the knowledge that whatever is in my body can be sent *out* of my body and does not have to drain into it. Meditation on expelling everything I have stored that is killing me—mostly memories and worries—feels proper. Pretty interesting. Maybe there is a bigger picture here: I don't have to take everything on and keep it inside, especially if it is sickening me.

Frank was very task-oriented in his meditations and came up with a bunch of work for me. First, I needed to change the core of my being! He said I needed to fall in love with three men: a poet, a dancer, and a lover.

"Couldn't that be you, Frank?" I ask. He has been all of those to me.
"I don't think so."
"And what will you be doing?"
"Keeping the home fires burning," he said.
"Well, all right, I'll look around." I was laughing but not amused. We both knew that picking up guys to dance, make love, or write poetry to me had not been one of my specialties.

———◇———

Everything is just irritating. Baaa. But my energy is OK, and I feel good. I'm overdue for some exercise, however. And I note that I'm hungry most of the time—even at night. This is sure slow, though, and speed is one of my virtues. About every hour I think, "Well, I could just get rid of the eye." But that makes no sense at all—the eye wouldn't stand a chance then. Another eye doc, actually a well-intentioned lad, suggested I have it poked out immediately.

"Your eye is half-dead. You don't see anything out of it. Why would you want to have a half-dead thing in your body?" he asked.

"But it is also half-alive—at least half." I think of some choice remarks about not seeing a horde of old dudes rushing to have their peepees whacked off when they only half work, but I think the better of it because I am enough of a source of irritation as it is. Odd thinking here, though, by George. I guess uteri after menopause might be considered at least half dead, and maybe we're schlepping around a whole lot of other dead and dying and atrophying detritus, like thymus glands and bad ears.

I have had a few "insights" (which I enclose in quotation marks, however, given the situation). In my meditations the last few days, I had been hearing "It is all connected. It is all connected." I recite this on the in-breath and out-breath. This meditation was done in the same room, on the same bed, where I had the "It is disconnected" dream after the night of wandering and the nosebleed from hell. Once the writing of this story is finished, I will recognize the connections and know what came loose. The faster I write, the quicker the answers will come, as if the writing itself were creating the metaphor, the book is the real world, and the daily routine is just a reflection, and maybe it is possible to write a life into a happy ending. Well, let's do it.

———◇———

I went back over the events of the root-canal infections, the low-grade fevers for a year or more, the dry eyes, and so forth. Then I began to think "what if" it was an infection, like the one around my tooth, and then I looked up the anatomy of the eye in *Behold Man,* a book of photographs of living tissues. Why did I wait so long to do this? Fear? This is the first thing I tell my patients to do, almost—take a look at the biology, the pathophysiology of their ailments. I discovered that the cornea does have a lymph drainage system. For two days (since imagining the debris oozing out of the cornea), I have had some stuff draining out. I had imaged the cornea's becoming porous, even tearing if necessary, to let out the junk. The cornea is tough and can repair itself.

I also remember my bout with sties in my left eye when I was eight years old, the magic age that all the dreamers had called to my atten-

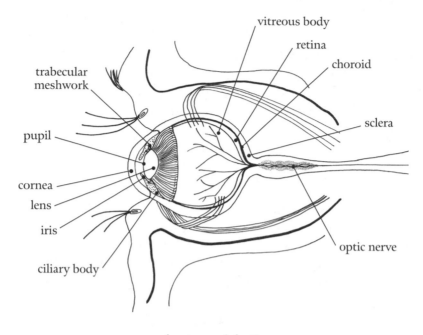

Anatomy of the Eye

tion. My grandmother took me to a doctor finally, and he quickly squeezed three of them. I yowled. The sties exploded and then got well.

Whatever it was that exploded this time did so throughout the area of the choroid. It did not have to burst through the retina necessarily. The choroid then becomes the iris. My iris was bloody and looked black—but I could see red underneath, especially in what I guess is the trabecular meshwork. All the mess is slowly going away, so someday we'll see what I've got left.

Matters of a Religious Nature

{February 5}

I AM OBSESSING, as I am prone to do, about how this story will end—and it *will* all come to some grand and glorious finale, I'm sure. I felt normal after a full day of writing. Today we worked out at the spa and went to town. In true do-it-yourself diagnostic fashion, I decided that the mess in my eye was protein deposits that were not being digested rapidly enough. So I upped the dose of enzymes and—for a couple of days, anyway—chewed papaya. I was also back on the full repertoire of supplements, including the megadose hit of energy and scintillating conversations during dinner with the Dosseys.

---◇---

I woke the next morning with the beginnings of the Headache from Hell and realize I must have screwed up my pH with so darn many acidic vitamins. That's probably what I've been doing all along when the Headache from Hell has struck. There is a book called *Who Goes First?* It is about scientists who have made their discoveries by experimenting on themselves. I plan to ask to be included if the book ever goes into a revised edition.

Ideas, they are a-churning. "Women, write down your thoughts, preserve your software, let history know what a woman does and thinks. Otherwise, generations to come can only recapitulate our failures; our lives and our wisdom go up the chimney in smoke. Write, dance, paint, speak—let your inner experience come alive." This is me quoting me.

Frank decided to go to church today, and I asked him why.

"It makes me feel good."

"I'll stay home. Church makes me feel terrible. Think I'll anoint myself with a little holy water and go sit on a rock."

Incidentally my holy water now is a mixture of waters from Lourdes (from Steve Wright), Saint Bridget's well in Ireland (Jo Wharton went there), Chalice Well in Glastonbury (from Judy Ostrow and me), and incense ash from the guru Sai Baba (from someone I do not know who became part of my healing web via the Internet). If this stuff doesn't do it, nothing will. It is turning slightly green.

I don't understand Frank's religious propensities. Last Easter we decided to go to church together. I picked an Episcopalian church, thinking the service would be ecumenical. Instead we got high fundamentalism. When we recited the Nicene Creed, I thought Frank was going to stroke out. He turned red and sweaty, and his collar looked too small. I guess Methodists from Texas don't do the creed, or he didn't remember it. Anyway, he said, "Let's get out of here." We went across the street to the well-known Catholic Church of Santa Fe, and he didn't improve any. My almost teetotaler of a husband said, "I need a drink, some real spirits." So we went to the famous La Fonda at the end of the Santa Fe Trail and ordered champagne.

Lately he's been going to one of the New Thought churches, which allow you to believe in just about anything, censor very little, are for the most part unconditionally positive, and where they invite him to talk.

I don't mean to make light of the religious thoughts, but here's where they trouble me. I have overheard him talking to one of his very fundamentalist Bible-church buddies in a voice that I don't recognize. The conversations are punctuated with "hallelujah," "yeah, brother," and phrases about the imminence of the Coming and the casting out of the Evil One (which I sometimes think means me and maybe a few of the girlfriends).

"Frank, why are you talking like that?" I finally asked.

"Just banter. Guy talk."

But I don't know, every alarm in my head started blaring. Who is this man, really? Did I help create this by something I did? Maybe he is a Jesus freak and won't tell me. Could it possibly be that my eclectic, free-form, slightly pagan and just a little Catholic spirituality with a feminist kick was a turnoff and forced him into this polemical position? Church had always made a community for Frank, until he met me; thereafter, dutifully or not, he had tended to remain as unchurched and free-spirited as I was, until just recently.

He always complained about the rages I flew into whenever he revealed some aspect of his interior life of which I was critical, and maybe that's why he kept the religious stuff secret from me. Yeah, I do rage— big-time and watch out—about once every two years, I admit it. It usually happens when I've had my fill of secrets. The last time I threw an entire set of glasses—not without just cause, of course—barely missing Frank and relishing every second of it, even the time it took me to clean up the mess. That performance could only have been carried off by the descendant of female Scandinavian warriors who chucked their spears into the thundering hordes while wearing metal breastplates and those gold hats with the horns.

I might well have thrown a hissy fit (another phrase I picked up in the south, and I might add, all that traveling as an army brat does expand your idiom) over the language I was overhearing about the Apocalypse. When gathered together, two or more fundamentalists of any persuasion are as dangerous as a pack of wild dogs, but maybe this was just the equivalent of religious locker-room talk. What do I know? Another item to be tucked away in my mental file cabinet for future reference.

Answered Prayers

{February 7}

TODAY I THOUGHT that if I could hear from my son, it would be important; my healing process could take a new twist. It has now been about three months since he's called. Please, God, let me hear from him.

Chase never acknowledged his Christmas presents. Last time he called, it was to Frank and for money. He is never absent from my thoughts: part of my brain is always with him, wondering, hoping. I wrote him a letter Thursday—first one ever that did not include a check. He usually calls when he is in bad trouble or in a very good place. No news means he is in the middle—nowhere. If he or any of the kids (Frank's or mine) are waiting for a trust fund before they start their lives in earnest, they'd better think again. It doesn't exist. We even forgot serious pension plans, an omission that's also weighing heavily on my mind.

The eye doesn't hurt at all but doesn't see any better either. "When my Vision returns, my vision will return" runs through my mind. Keep writing. Write of life to save life. Today I also thought of the true story of "Martha," whose journal became the book *O Rugged Land of Gold*. Long story, but she was a very young woman, stranded on an island in Alaska by an early winter, and an avalanche injured her severely. Her prospector husband had left to get supplies and was unable to return. She was pregnant and had never witnessed the birth of anything, not even a cat. She wrote and wrote on every usable scrap in the cabin, even during labor, to keep her mind off things she knew nothing about and to save her own life.

I went over in my head, and then with Frank, just how much time the Thing had cost him. Debits and credits. Surely he had learned something more about using alternative methods in the treatment of cancer, and this should be a credit. Oh, yes, I'm getting better. I'm bitching again.

My good news is that Elsa, an ophthalmologist in our training two years ago, has contacted me. Now that I have her on E-mail, at least I have an eye person who will listen to the story and give me some imagery. Elsa is retired and practicing Reiki, a method of energy healing. Here's the message I got from her after asking about imagery:

> Regarding Reiki: Given your schedule and my few obligations over the next two weeks, I suggest that at about 3:00 P.M. each day you find a comfortable spot for relaxing and I will send the Reiki healing from 3:00 to 3:15 P.M. each day except Saturday, February 12, when I'll send at about 10:00 A.M. If you're tied up with something, that's OK. These things work in mysterious ways, which are not necessarily time-related. Any feedback you might have is welcome, particularly after several days. And of course, if you sense some discomfort with this, I know you'll let me know ASAP. Some of the Reiki teachings suggest that some people have some discomfort initially. That has not been a problem in my experience.
>
> Regarding imagery for your eye: I do have concerns about simply doing imaging to clear the inflammatory response. Sometimes the inciting agent continues to exist. Other times it may be gone but the inflammation continues. If there is still original abnormal tissue, whatever it may be, that needs healing, physiologically there would still need to be increased capillary permeability to allow lymphocytes and chemical mediators to reach the site of concern. I know you have the knowledge and wisdom for appropriate imagery. With that stated, what I would recommend to an inexperienced person would be to suggest to that inner healing wisdom that *if* all the abnormal tissue has been taken care of and there is

no further need for an inflammatory response, that all the capillaries in the uveal tract (the choroid, which is just beneath the retina, ciliary body, and iris) and retina return to their normal state of impermeability, except for what is necessary to normally nourish the eye. The inflammatory cells and protein will gradually clear through blood vessels and the trabecular meshwork, which is in the shape of a circle where the iris meets the sclera as you visualize the front of the eye. It would be helpful to image the clearing in the trabecular meshwork to be gradual so as not to clog the meshwork, which could cause an increase in the intraocular pressure and pain. Any fibrotic tissue that is not needed for walling off the origi-nal abnormal tissue could also be visualized as gradually break-ing down.

I am interested in your image of the Thing exploding. I'm not sure how to think about that physiologically. Could it be that the sense of an explosion was the inflammatory reaction? And the de-bris you've seen is actually inflammatory debris?

Regarding vision: The "party line" would be that there is proba-bly disruption through fibrosis and possibly growth of new vessels as a healing response of the retinal structure—rods and cones and their connections—that would create a problem for the return of vision. So again imaging the dissolution of unneeded fibrous tissue and blood vessels would be appropriate, along with a realignment of the rods and cones.

Hopefully this is helpful to you. Sometimes I find myself getting caught up in wanting to have the anatomy and physiology and im-munology absolutely accurate. I believe that there is a higher force and wisdom that I can trust if my intent is there. As I have come to that place, I have felt a great relief. That is not to say I should slough off and not care and not try. But in the end I know I am turning this over to a greater power than myself.

Elsa confirmed my imagery and encouraged my patience. I think the Thing is gone, but then again, I never knew it was there in the first place. I also believe that any systemic problem is gone. Elsa has come into my life at just the perfect time, as have so many, and her words are like gold for my healing.

Despite Elsa's E-mail, I couldn't get settled enough to write nor tired enough to sleep. I drove out to Espanola for rock for the gardens and realized that I just couldn't see—not necessarily a bad thing, but so much light was coming in that I had to squint to get depth perception. When I got home, I just didn't know how to feel better, so I took a "coffee break," a sauna, and a bath. My mistletoe arrived, so I shot up.

I prayed for my son to call. I had reached my limit and was about to either phone the doctor or the police or go out to California myself.

After three months of silence, as if he had heard my desperation, Chase called—on Frank's line. I have no idea where he was calling from, but it was collect. He told Frank he had learned how to control the Voices. He told me two Chinese parables, which I didn't understand and asked him to write down for me. They seemed to be about an underdog who realized he'd had at least one day when he didn't get kicked. He said he was going to try to find a job the next day. I decided to drive to California to do rescue work, then changed my mind, as usual, when the reality of driving such a distance alone stared me in the face.

We call the builder over to begin plans for the caretaker's casita. This is a major direction and a new era for us: we need extra space. I don't want anyone living under our large roof, but we do need help with the puppies, the house, and the grounds. Not only that, I'm just plain lonely in the mud palace. I need a wife or a personal assistant or a bunch of friends around.

As I reread all this writing, I'm realizing how much anger is being expressed, and I promise myself that I'll edit it out to make it sound more uplifting, which I do. Some.

Another helpful E-mail from Elsa:

> Thanks for taking the time to share your amazing experience! It sounds like you've been to the Underworld and back. Knowing about the initiation that shamans go through, I'm wondering where this will lead you.
>
> Your writing and sharing of this experience is really important. It will give courage to others in this society who may have had a similar experience but are reluctant to share it. It is critical to make this knowledge public, particularly from someone with your academic credentials, if we are going to reach new planes or levels of reality for healing and living.

In response to a few questions in your E-mail—am thinking that the circle around the pupil that looked bloody could have either been some hemorrhage on the iris or, if the circle was actually where the cornea meets the sclera (the limbus), which is what I think you're describing, there are perilimbal vessels that may selectively dilate and become engorged when there is uveitis. Subjectively it appears to be the area where the iris meets the sclera, since the cornea is normally transparent. Regarding whether or not the eye wants to try to see—I think wearing a patch is optional. Part of the health of the surface of the eye is maintained by the blinking of the lids, so I would discourage your having it patched closed.

P.S. Jeanne, I know you have a breadth of scientific knowledge that may make my explanations too simple and unnecessary. But I put them out anyway.

She flattered me. I had remained blissfully ignorant of the physiology of the eye until just a few days ago.

———◇———

I'm beginning to realize something. When I'm writing this stuff, it's as if I were going through it all over again. There is no relief. I'm getting to the tough parts now. This is all about cleaning up my life. Either I will or I won't. Having time to do this with some consciousness is a fortunate gift.

———◇———

Frank and I did our morning ritual of making coffee and bringing it back to bed for about twenty minutes of conversation. Such a truly loving, supportive time in the winter. When it gets warm, we'll guzzle the coffee and then talk while we walk these puppies. They are getting hard to manage, don't mind, and chew on everything in sight, including the hoses and the screen doors. Today we talked about our landscaping, our dreams from the night before. We both have airplane dreams. He's rushing to catch one, and I can't find my tickets.

In the afternoon the eye did a weird thing. Very red, no pain. I imagine the blood vessels have dilated to allow it to drain, and I did about one and a half hours' meditation on this idea. That much meditation time is a miracle, since twenty minutes used to stretch my capacity for staying still and remaining focused.

Did mistletoe injections—trusting that if inflammation was needed, it would happen. Carl called to check in. Frank phoned from work just to see how my day was going. This was a new pattern for him, which I didn't understand but deeply appreciated.

This from Elsa:

> The location of the trabecular meshwork is where the iris and cornea meet, so it is circular as one looks at the eye. It is not accessible to view unless a special lens is placed on the cornea. Microscopically it looks like fenestrated intertwining sheets of connective tissue with mainly collagen and some elastic fibers and lined by endothelial cells. These channels eventually connect with a larger opening called Schlemm's canal, which drains into various venous channels and into the orbital veins. The aqueous humor [the clear fluid that circulates in the space between the lens and the cornea] and anything suspended in it, like cells and protein, drain through the meshwork, so it is draining from inside to outside the eye via the venous system. Hope this helps.
>
> Am continuing the Reiki healing sessions for now. I would share with you that these are highly energetic times for me, which I believe has to do with the recipient. Thanks for this opportunity. I will continue until you advise me otherwise or until you begin your traveling, if that seems best.

Valentine

{February 13}

FRANK HAS LEFT for Dallas today, and I'm glad because I can get some more writing done.

On Friday he tiptoed in the door (but I caught him) carrying a bouquet of bright orange roses and handmade turquoise earrings. Early Valentine's Day. Yesterday, Saturday, we played, shopped, stuffed ourselves with junk food, watched a bunch of videos and snow flurries outside, made margaritas and chili, wrestled with the pups, and stayed in bed from three in the afternoon until morning. I gave him his Valentine gift—two wolves carved out of white stone and tied together with brown twine. They were from a Zuni craftsman and symbolized "the two as one."

I have this theory that couples make love the way they dance together. We danced with grace from time and experience and the pleasure of moving to music. We had only a few cocreated steps, but we did them very well.

On Valentine's weekend, the time of the celebration of love, nothing was different and everything was. I was a sleepwalker who had awakened in a dark and nameless place. Was he someone different, somewhere else, or was he no one? He seemed not to know me either; I could have been anyone or no one, and I felt as if I'd been rendered anonymous. Was he, too, a sleepwalker, and was I the only one awake—and, by the way, how long had this been going on? I didn't know.

I tried to talk about it, and Frank vaguely referred to a diversion of our energies. I didn't know what that meant. Could it be that having a Grim Reaper diagnosis isn't sexy? That has been known to happen in the annals of the history of disease. Frank firmly maintained that I had been misdiagnosed—that I had something, but it was not grim. I had to stash this experience in the mental file cabinet, because I couldn't do anything about it right then.

With all that said, we've been cuddling again at night, and I am grateful for the extended physical contact. For months he has huddled on his side of the bed, and he hurts so much of the time that I have tried to stay away so I don't jar him or put pressure on a sore joint.

Last night, in the middle of the night, he had another gout attack. This has been happening more often than not. They say gout is the equivalent of childbirth pain, and it's mostly men who have gout. I don't doubt it hurts, though. He walked as if he was in pain all the time. I did some massage on his back and legs and felt blocks of vital energy. Hot here, cold there, but heat is not necessarily energy. We may need to request home health care for the two of us if this keeps up.

Anyway, the weekend had been our idea of a good time, more or less. We've made plans for a fountain on a foundation of pink quartz, which is really a glorified drinking bowl for the dogs. The cost of these animals is now in the thousands, and I'm afraid to open the bill from the landscaper. Yes, I have something to live for: I want to see these guys grow up.

Toward the end of January, I had started using a meditation that Carl suggested. Basically it is like mindfulness meditations. You take in energy and healing and just let them gravitate to wherever they need to go. "In a childlike way," you give away any troubles or pain. I fed all my negative thoughts to wolves.

Or I'd use the nineteen-ribbon thing from Steve's dream, imagining nineteen ribbons streaming from my eye, counting each one. Some led to my brain, others to outer space. I imagined each one clear, clean, connected to where it needed to be.

Yesterday—and this is an important piece—I mentioned to Frank that the Thing was thinning out in wedge shapes. Like pieces being cut from a pie. I can see about four pieces or wedges. He said he remembered a study on eardrums at the medical school where he worked. At that time they would either puncture kids' eardrums to insert drains or let the eardrums burst on their own and drain naturally. When they punctured the eardrums, scar tissue was a problem, as was healing. When they allowed the eardrums to burst by themselves, they healed in wedge shapes. It must have had something to do with maintaining pressure inside an organ. This will be added to my imagery. The cold bothered my eye outside today, and it got milky-looking. But today I absolutely knew it was getting well, molecule by molecule.

Work from my several day jobs is piling up, I have other writing to do, the house is a mess, and I am flat-out fatigued from reconstructing the entire eye journey. When the book is finished, a chapter in my life will close, and I am anxious for that to happen because I want to see how it ends.

———◇———

I set my intention for the week to get some remarkable feedback from the eye. No luck. It is taking its own sweet time.

Frank said this writing was me doing psychotherapy on myself in order to achieve catharsis. That kind of talk is what keeps me from being a very enthusiastic member of my own profession and leaves me wishing I could go into retail. Maybe he's right, but those seem like such small, dismissive words for what is actually an attempt to discover my story, reinvent myself back into something that will survive. For me the writing is a revelatory experience, and almost each day one mysterious piece of the puzzle falls into place. Other days it is just tedious shit.

———◇———

A little retrospective eye observation. All sinus drainage from the eye stopped about ten days ago—for the first time since summer. Also, I've had no skin reaction to this series of mistletoe—not even a red mark. I changed from mistletoe grown on oak trees to a preparation from mistletoe harvested from apple trees, which is more typically prescribed for women. God forbid, maybe I need the man-size dose to get a reaction.

———◇———

I felt very sick last night. It could be the writing—hit some heavy parts—or that I didn't eat all day on Valentine's Day or that Chase called again. He said he had an intuition he needed to contact me, just to see how I was doing.

Elsa's advice that the complexity of the eye and what it went through is going to require an equally complex and long healing time stays with me. Patience. My impatience runs through this writing. Get on with it, say I.

Flowers fell out of my journal this morning. I remember having picked them at the Chalice Well in Glastonbury. Jo Wharton, my Dallas friend, sent me a card from Ireland, which I received today. She took my picture to Saint Bridget's well last week and did prayers for the return of my vision. A day of holy wells!

The symptoms of the past November (of which I was writing) returned today. And of course. Flashbacks.

I spoke with Jonathan Green at Shambhala Publications, and he voiced his amazement at how the symbolic and mythic nature of my life was becoming so prominent and important. "I have only had glimpses in my own life of this, and it is something to command attention." We spoke of Saint Lucy, the patron of vision on the cover of my book *Woman as Healer*. He said, "Go figure." Shambhala had chosen the cover, not I.

Mara Jan called. She had received my records and pictures of my eye. We requested the records at the time she accompanied me to the offices of one of the eye docs, where I underwent the most gruesome series of tests. I had signed releases for all of them and asked that the results be mailed. None were until we pressed the issue last week, nearly six months later. I did not yet want to look at them. She was astonished that the pictures looked like the lightning flashes we had seen during the storm in Marin County, when I began the shamanic trek with Michael Harner. I went back over my thoughts and recaptured the number of times lightning has been part of this theme—lightning storms, Lightning Beaver, lightning behind the eye, dreams of lightning striking me in the garden. Must mean something.

Dreamer

{February 17}

LEE LAWSON REMINDED ME of the dream she had about me two years ago, which neither I nor quite a few other people will ever forget, since it was in a newsletter published by the Institute of Noetic Sciences (IONS). I was scheduled to give a keynote lecture in Kansas City on the Fourth of July at the IONS conference, timed between my near-death experience in the dental chair and the revenge of the black widows. The talk was on "Uncommon Bonds," and I was focusing on the transpersonal relationship some people have with one another, relationships that defy the bounds of time and space. I always use slides of Lee's art when I give this talk, because she has painted splendid pictures of humans in relationship.

Lee felt she needed to get the dream information to me quickly and before I left for Kansas City. She had dreamed I was in a situation in which fire alarms began to go off. Emergencies were repeatedly announced. There appeared to be grave danger. But she wanted me to know that it would turn out to be a false alarm. Everything would be fine.

At 7:00 in the morning, the fire alarms started to go off in the hotel. For real. The elevators stopped. I got trapped on the first floor at breakfast, with my notes and slides on the twenty-second floor. It reminded me of the *Titanic*. People were scrambling up and down the emergency exits, and it was the Fourth of July so about half the employees had called in "sick," which added to the chaos. I tried to run up the stairs

(I really needed my slides and notes; this was a virgin talk), and by the eighth floor I just couldn't keep going up the stifling, hot stairs in my medium-high heels. A strong, brave conference volunteer ran the rest of the way up, went into my room, and retrieved what I needed.

As I was showing Lee's slides and talking about the uncommon bond she and I share, a voice came on the loudspeaker telling us all to proceed quickly to the emergency exits and evacuate the room. The voice came on again and again, and I had to quit talking each time. The audience and I laughed nervously for a while, and then I would just stop talking during the sirens and resume when they quit. Almost the moment I finished the lecture, another voice came on the loudspeaker and said, sorry, it was all just a false alarm.

Lee thinks this past year has been like that for me—a series of emergencies that would turn out to be false alarms. A double-duty dream.

I don't know what auspicious day this is, but there is a full moon. I am glad to be alive. Really. My son called again just to say, "I love you, Mom."

"Do we need to finish up our business? You know, when people love each other as much as we do, things sometimes get all twisted up."

"No, Mom. I'm fine. We're fine. I used to have some problems with our relationship, but it's OK now."

Whatever this Eye Thing is, I can live with it. And I wouldn't trade one moment of this precious passage for anything.

Unfinished Business

{February 22}

I HAVE RECENTLY been asking myself, "Would I be doing this now (whatever "this" is that I'm doing during any given inquiry) if I knew that my life, as I know it, might end soon?" I've never given an affirmative answer until just the last couple of months. Absolutely. Why didn't I think of this before the urgency, the slight (oh, so slight) disability of my whole if slightly aging self? Because I just didn't.

Working with people who had cancer had taught me well, I thought, because for many of them there was no bullshit, no pettiness, and what was cream rose to the top. They mostly got their priorities straight. I really did learn from them, but life got out of hand, it seems.

But yes, I would do as I am doing now—writing, trying to lay down a trail for others to follow (including the manure I've stepped in), and finishing business.

There is one very old chunk of unfinished business, which has been with me almost forever—a closure that was never made honorable with a person who was one of the epiphanies in my own young life. Remember the three guys who counted? Two of them were my husbands. The other was Tony, my almost husband and first love. I married, instead, the man who I thought would be better able to go with me to where I needed to go in life (having no clue, mind you, where that might be).

Today Tony E-mailed me: "You've been haunting me for forty years. I need to make an apology. Overreacting has been my major problem, and I overreacted."

At first I didn't understand. I was the one who needed to apologize, and I'd been looking for him in telephone books in every city in the world. He'd gone to Vietnam twice, and I'd guessed he was dead. I checked the names on the Wall, and his was not among them, though. So here we go. A classic example of "unfinished business" has magically appeared.

He was captain of the football team, and I was head cheerleader. In our senior year I was homecoming queen, and he was my escort. The live band played "Autumn Leaves" and "Ebb Tide" while we swirled away in the center of the ballroom. I wore purple velvet and lace and had made the dress and matching gloves myself. Having taken eight semesters of home economics, I could make nearly anything of a domestic nature.

It just doesn't get much better than that. At least then, it didn't. The American Dream of the fifties. He gave me a little diamond ring, and then he moved away. You move all the time when you're an army brat, even if it means leaving high school in your senior year. He showed up on my front steps the day I was leaving Germany to return to the United States in 1962. Only problem, I was already in the car with Mel. The three of us spent a weekend and not exactly together. We had a schedule. I got the pleasure of one's company for two hours, and then the other one. My family was staying in some dreadful transit hotel in Frankfurt, and we'd sent our luggage ahead but the plane was delayed. I had to wash my underwear out at night, and it never got quite dry. You wore girdles then (even at ninety-eight pounds) to keep your stockings up. One whole weekend in a wet girdle.

Mel and Tony stayed in the same room at night—which I will never understand, except neither of them had any money, and neither of them remembers much about those nights. The future of my life was hanging in the balance—and so was theirs. The one I loved better was the one I was *not* with. That's all I can say. I saw Tony last. Well, there was a little more to it: Mel was slightly more ambitious, or at least I thought so. Tony then looked like a cross between Marlon Brando and Paul Newman (who are both old now, but so are we). Mel looked like Desi Arnaz and still does a little. ("You married Desi, not Marlon?!" my friend Fleur Green yelped.)

205

Yes, indeed. This is a time for endings and beginnings. Makes me think of T. S. Eliot:

> What we call the beginning is often the end
> And to make an end is to make a beginning.
> The end is where we start from.

———◇———

Gar Hildebrand called again, just checking up on me. He used to be the research director of the Gerson Institute and is now doing some work investigating case results from some of the alternative centers around the world. I helped Gar get his research published in the *Alternative Therapies* journal. He probably knows as much about melanoma as anyone. The Gerson methods seem to work best for that condition, and that's what his article was about.

I told him, with some temerity, about the eye attack and my current status of aliveness. He reminded me about John, a man we both know who had a spontaneous remission right there in front of Gar. John had had a huge tumor under his arm, which swelled to twice its size, and it caused indescribable pain. Redness and bruising spread around his back and sides. Then there was a moment of transcendence, the pain changed character, and within two months the tumor completely disappeared, leaving not even a scar. Gar was reasonably convinced that this is what had happened to me.

"What else could it be?" I asked.

"Nothing," he said. "You're not going in the 'expected' direction but the unexpected." I asked about the pain, and he said when a large amount of tumor necrosis factor (TNF) is released, it's painful. Now things were starting to make sense. In November I was in deadly shock. The cold fire.

"If anyone could have a spontaneous remission, it would be you." I suppose this is true. Both he and I knew there is nothing spontaneous about any remission. Remissions happen on the crest of the hardest work you can ever perform—the work of changing your life. He quoted a passage from *The Cloud of Unknowing* (written by a mystic back when) and from Rudolf Steiner, the mistletoe man. I do find it so very intriguing that poetry and pearls of spiritual wisdom are interspersed with medical information by so many who have extended their help.

Gar said that the garbage in my eye was probably protein and that the body would get rid of it sooner or later. I was wishing sooner. He was my man of the day.

And More Dream Helpers

{February 25}

FRANK AND I TRAVELED to Indiana to teach our year-long training at Oakwood Farm Retreat Center, our program on health. I love these folks—Midwestern, nonjaded, humorous, and seriously spiritual. They were the first to learn of my "condition" through a public disclosure, and they were the ones whom Frank taught alone last November, while I was spiking fevers, or whatever they were, from the eye attack.

The group had done a "dream helper" session on me February 18. Through E-mail communication, they all chose the night to dream of my healing. That night I thought bugs were in the bed and crawling around on me and finally just got up and sat in a chair. I had forgotten it was dream night, actually, but being the target of some heavy-duty transpersonal images could make you feel as if you needed to scratch.

About fifteen members of the group described their dreams, and we audiotaped the discussion. The variety and complexity of the dreams were astonishing. Quite a few were simply incomprehensible, and I will try to redream them—take the images into my dream world and find out what they might mean.

One very proper lady dreamed that she was waiting for a bus and many kept passing her by. She said, "Oh, fuck, I'll take a taxi." She never says "Oh, fuck." I do, though, and that is pretty much what I said after modern medicine and a few other folks kept passing me by. And I rode by myself in a taxi. All the dreams had a happy ending or at least a neutral one. Would they have told me if they'd seen me in an urn? I wonder. One dreamer actually described the view outside my bedroom window, the quartz mountain at the back of the house. Some had visions in the waking state. One woman described a vision in which *my* vision was partly restored. Nerves had been compressed by the pressure of the explosion in November and would not return unless the original blueprint was reformulated. That is entirely possible and what I believe also. What's amazing (and it shouldn't be) is that (1) so many people decided to dedicate a night to dreaming about me, and (2) most of them had relevant dreams.

Dwight Judy, our host, dreamed of a box with the word *teaching* in it and lots of space around. Teaching alone. The kidney-shaped tumor thing also shriveled up. This made sense. I needed to get off my bitchin' duff and get back to teaching in all its many forms—especially now that I had some new material.

Frank drew his dream on a yellow sticky pad and said I was supposed to eat the page. I'm looking at it as I write, wondering how to get it down the hatch. The symbols he drew were a bird; feathers; "aol," as if it were some Internet communication; triangles; an open mouth; arrows; and the numbers 84 and 58. A sticky note doesn't chew, dissolve, or go down; it sits there and expands. I asked Frank to eat a corner of it just so he could understand what I was up against.

David, a member of the group who was enjoying a fairly miraculous state of health after a diagnosis of prostate cancer, dreamed the words of an ancient Irish hymn:

> Be Thou my vision,
> O Lord of my heart;
> Naught be all else to me,
> Save that Thou art.
> Thou my best thought,
> By day or by night,
> Waking or sleeping,
> Thy presence my light.

Oakwood has been where major turning points in our lives were sparked or at least facilitated. During the last, or fourth, phase of the training, I always talked about the healing power of relationships. Usually I would use Frank's heart attack as an example, describe the challenges I faced as a support person, and funny it up a bit. It hadn't been humorous, though; it had been dreadful, every second of it, and the recovery period had been even worse.

This time in Indiana, I got to use me and what support I got as the example and went over some of the stories in this book. Several members of the group requested that Frank share his experiences also.

"Hoo-boy," I thought, "no telling what he'll say, because he's never spoken a word about this to me or anyone else that I know of."

He explained, "Jeanne and I are both Aries, and everyone predicted we would kill each other within three months after we were married." We're stubborn rams, I guess he meant. I don't think we even fight decently. I bark and throw; he ducks and retreats into a cave of silence or just leaves. That's it. End of fight.

"Everyone needs someone to go up against, to fight with. I provided that for Jeanne." Silence.

I tried to calm the collective shudder. "Frank actually did much more than provide me with someone to go up against," I told the group. "He went grocery shopping, ran errands, and even came home occasionally to fix lunch when he knew I was having a bad day."

Someone in the group asked how I felt about needing someone to fight with for support. What can you say?

"Being angry is certainly more energizing than being depressed," I answered. No point in letting the group do therapy on us.

Then Frank volunteered information about the time deal: "I had to draw my own boundaries during this whole thing. Jeanne wanted to stop everything we were doing and go away someplace for six months and just concentrate on each other. I had to tell her that I just couldn't leave my own life to do that sort of thing."

"But you really didn't believe she was going to die, did you?" asked David. David and his wife (also in the group) were in their seventies, a beautiful couple, brilliant and well-heeled, who were taking turns caring for each other during their golden years.

Frank laughed and said, "No, of course not. She's misdiagnosed." And I, of course, am still hoping he was correct.

Last summer I had asked him to go away with me. I said, "I know I could get well if we went off to Greece or someplace for six months and focused on healing." What I really meant was, "I do not believe I can regain my vision in the same environment where there is so much stress and tension and where the work is relentless. You are the most important person in my life, and if I go away, I do not want to leave you. And I hope you love me enough to agree." I've never been to Greece, and the place was not the point.

Sometimes I have to tell Frank what I need, and it pisses me off royally that I need something, number one, and that he can't figure it out without my telling him, number two. Mostly it is number two.

Relationship Ruminations

{February 26}

OH, GAWD. The worst of the worst. Last night I injured my other eye—the reasonably good one. It felt as if I scratched my cornea, but I think I cooked it. At night I nearly freeze because my body is closer to the open window, so I sleep with a hot-water bottle. I must have had my face on it. If you've ever injured a cornea, you know where nine-tenths of your pain receptors are, regardless of what the textbooks say. Plus, I couldn't see. That's why you don't casually let someone zap an eye. You need at least one, and removal makes you very vulnerable. Chugalug, down go the anti-inflammatories, the pain meds. Bummer. I still can't see distinctly today. Both eyes look the same. I knew it, someone has been praying for both my eyes to be the same.

I stayed in bed for a couple of hours while Frank went grocery shopping. During my meditation I heard the word *dragmailer,* having no clue what it meant, and also had the spontaneous image of a snake poised to strike in my left eye. I took that as a good sign—transformation, DNA, which looks snakelike, repairing itself. No point in thinking anything negative right now.

Frank was warm and present and especially nice today. "Frank, I really don't need you to fight with me. I've got the American Medical Association and my mother, and that's a handful. I just need you to cuddle, take me out to dinner, tell me everything is going to be all right." Man, I don't get it. Why would I need someone to fight with? I am feeling terrible, have been given the equivalent of a death sentence, and all I want to do is tuck myself under the covers and try to figure out where I go from here.

———◇———

Chase called today. Good thing one of the girlfriends gave me the "tough-love" lecture last week. I was braced. He wants to come out here and start his life over. Things aren't going well. His car has been impounded for not being registered, and he's got a charge against him—"assault on a police officer," no less. But I'm assured it is a misdemeanor and only involves paying a small fine. He needs money— twelve hundred dollars, to be exact—to get his car out, registered, pay his fine for assault, and so on. Then he'll be right on out to Santa Fe. He's clean and sober, he says, and that counts for something.

I'm thinking how wonderful it would be to give him a fresh start. He's so smart, so talented, so loving when he's not using. We're going to turn part of the garage into a small apartment, and he could live there. He could drive me places where I'm not sure I could hit the parking space. He could find a job, be treated by our psychiatrist friends at the state hospital, get well. Maybe he just needs to get out of California, needs his mother. I can cook hearty soups and stews and help put meat on his fragile bones. He could sleep in a good, clean bed and hear the night animal sounds and see the moon glisten on the active mountain. God, I love that boy.

Too familiar. I remember this. So I make stipulations. He can't bring his pit bull. (Now I ask, does that sound unreasonable?) "What, not bring Misty? Well, if you say so, I'll leave her here." He can't come until the apartment in the garage is finished—maybe May. He needs to find a job in California and work for a couple of months to show us he can hold down a job. And we can't send the money. And he'll need to get treatment once he's here. Two or three more calls to talk to Frank about "things" that I have been exempted from hearing. Finally we said, "No more calls" tonight, and he agreed to try to find another way to get his car out of hock.

You can't just throw away a kid. You can't give up on him, even if he is thirty-one years old. But nothing has swayed Chase from this lifestyle. He is lovable, and he's worn us all out. There is always hope, though. Maybe next time.

213

———◇———

Two days later I E-mailed Tony, telling him I appreciated the opportunity to catch up and wanted to do it in a way that would be appropriate for him. Bam. Bam. More E-mail. He was elated, couldn't concentrate, and focused on me while he was bowling and couldn't remember his score. I must admit a little preoccupation, because I'm a curious woman and was happy to remember some of the most innocent, joyful days of my life. Lightning Beaver days. Maybe that's what this was about—remembered joy. Tony had a series of questions for me, saying he was going crazy trying to read between my lines. I would need to be clearer and skip the babble of the sensitive New Age woman.

Mainly, Tony asked, would my husband be threatened if we established some communication? Not likely, thought I. Not after he spent five years (that I know of) intensely involved with a married woman with grown children who answered telephones for a living. He was infatuated with her, he said, because she led a conventional life, and he was "exploring the archetype of a plain woman." I was handicapped by my own femininity and the desire to live a full, and therefore complicated, life. Plain and ordinary were grounds upon which I could not compete. "Are you looking for a new wife?" I frequently inquired.

"No, you keep misunderstanding me. I'm looking for a new life. I'm wondering what it would be like for us to live a simpler life."

Well, anyway, those were our bad years, and whether he was looking for a new wife, I don't know, but he was certainly looking for a new life. Frank disliked California and most Californians and longed to be closer to his children and later his grandchildren, his Texas culture, and what he called "true home." He quit his job as president of the Institute of Transpersonal Psychology in Menlo Park two months after his inauguration in 1990 and never really found a professional niche. In 1995 he had a heart attack—one way to end it all—and survived to move to New Mexico, slightly closer to his heart's desires.

Guess I'll explore another archetype with an old friend, if that's what you want to call it. Frank says he thinks it's a good idea to get reacquainted with old friends, and he gets threatened by very little that I do. Course I don't do much of anything except love a lot of men who feel like my brothers. Tony wanted a real telephone call, but we needed to work around his bowling nights. Jeanne the Queen has never been in a bowling alley and doesn't know anyone who has except Mo, who bowled in a league when her girls were young. I'll ask Mo about this when she gets back from wherever she's gone. She did tell me you couldn't buy bowling shirts in Neiman Marcus and had to go to J. C. Penney. I wonder whether bowlers do Tantric sex. Probably no more often than Texans, and Mo says that's because you can't do Tantric in a truck.

Eye check. The sorta good eye has about returned, but I do have to keep adjusting my glasses. The eye is no longer red; it's barely pink. It is neither swollen nor snotty. The light coming in is really overwhelming, and today I probably could not drive unless I squinted to shut out the light. And, I must remember to add, in Indiana my appetite was ferocious. I ate that midwestern food like a starved little pig. Am still wondering where the appetite went for a couple of months. Maybe the tumor necrosis factor was being liberated into my whole body—it causes cachexia (lack of appetite)—or maybe I had the flu (everybody else did), or maybe I was just scared to death.

I am doing enzymes and whatever supplement my intuitive hand lands on. Swing the pendulum, pick a pill. Mistletoe tomorrow.

As I'm writing, a blizzard is moving in. The windows are shaking from the wind, and the pups are cowering. Energy is gathering on the sacred mountain. Time to shut down the computer. The weather always plays like an orchestra behind my life, so things are blowing and going, extreme conditions for Santa Fe.

This thing with number one may be getting out of hand. Tony received my pictures. I'd sent him the ones from the photo shoot of "Santa Fe Originals—Women Who Broke the Mold," so they were pretty darn good.

"Didn't sleep a wink last night. I placed the new pictures beside the eight-by-ten school photo of you. If someone had seen me, they would have thought I had a serious mental problem. I just sat there smiling and analyzing every detail. God, you are gorgeous! Stared into your eyes and felt a warmth similar to what I felt so long ago. Up to now your pictures left a cold, hollow feeling in my chest. Now I see and feel joy."

Then he tells me the weirdest thing. He lost all his stuff when his dad sold his own house, including everything in it, bought a motor home, and went to Tucson. When his dad died in 1988, he left Tony's yearbook and the picture of me in the trunk of a 1959 Edsel. Tony drove out to pick up the car and was so devastated by the memories, he broke down, checked into a motel, and called his daughter, whom he knew would understand.

We're talking forty years here. I can't get my mind around all this. I'm dragging my feet. Don't want to lead Tony down a path of no return, but it sounds as though he's already been there. After me neither of his marriages was quite right, he said.

I got his picture in the mail. His Cherokee blood is very obvious now. He looks like a "breed," as they call themselves, just like Grandfather Raven and Rolling Thunder, two very blue-eyed medicine men.

The girlfriends have all checked in, and eye feels normal. Color is nearly normal. No aches, no pains. Did not start the mistletoe series. Seem to keep forgetting it. Plenty of enzymes, pills for the nurturance of the eye, luteins, s-adenosyl-methionine (SAMe), and coenzyme Q10 (CoQ10). I slept horribly last night. Moved to another room. Can't even blame it on the puppies. Maybe I am just not tired anymore.

How much longer, dear God, till the light returns full blast? Am I ready to let the Thing go? Here's the deal: Life perked up after the Thing announced itself. Sheer terror is better than sheer boredom. The world shifted on its axis. When the light returns (notice I say when, not if), I've got more challenges on my hands: (1) a life to plan and (2) a little confrontation with the medical system. Now this is predictable. My situation will turn out to be either a misdiagnosis (in which case they were all pretty hasty to recommend slicing it out) or me imagining that I'm well. I will probably have some visual loss for a time until I can figure out how to fix it. The sonograms may look like crap for a long time. So those are pretty big items on my agenda. And (3) I need to sort through everything that has been accumulating in the mental file cabinet. But not now.

Frank and I went out for our midweek dinner—red meat at Steaksmith down the road. I told him about the day and Tony. His eyes lit up at the mention of an Edsel. Then he told me I must be very concrete in this situation—be the real me, and then any illusions will vanish. He had feelings, he said, for a college sweetheart for fifteen years after his marriage to Gloria. The feelings dissolved when he called her. She had a bunch of kids, yelled in a twang like a banshee, and he immediately remembered all the things he didn't like about her. What he had liked best was that she passed out every time she had an orgasm. Imagine that in the back seat of a 1956 Chevy. First he thought she was dead and dressed her to take her to the emergency room or the morgue, but she woke up. Hard to forget a girl like that.

I said, "But Tony's loved me all these years. That's something. All I ever wanted was someone to love me, just me, unconditionally, no matter what. I didn't ask for all this career business. Remember, I majored in home economics in high school so I could be the perfect wife and mother."

Tony said that every relationship he'd had since me was "almost but not quite OK." Frank goes through some bullshit about that's how all men are affected by me, but that's part of his mating dance, and I don't believe it for a minute.

"That's how I love you," Frank says.

"You've never said that."

"Yes, I have. I told you that you were the omega one. There would be no women after you. It would not be possible."

"Tony says I am gorgeous."

"I say that all the time." Not really, but he has increased his admiration lately, either because he thinks there is competition or because I'm sprucing up out of my deathbed. He never once mentioned that I was the omega one and the gorgeous one during those many months of healing.

I'm thinking now, you wouldn't invest your time in one person (me) if you thought she was fading away into Glory and twelve weeks might be asking a little too much. You would be trying to protect yourself, keep a life going. Basic survival instincts. The office staff and the needy women patients who knock on his door and call him at all hours of the night and day are not likely to be ignored, any more than they are now. Well, let me think about this, because I'm beginning to wonder whether Frank's reluctance to invest more than twelve weeks in my "process," as he calls it, is a survival strategy in case I should be resting in peace shortly. Omega one I do not think I am.

If I graduate into the Beyond, at least I've left him some IRAs and a big mud palace, and he can survive forever if he doesn't go overboard and buy a bunch of toys. Why am I thinking these morbid thoughts? What if he dies and I cannot work? I am getting back to the thing about the pension plan—which I do not have, and Frank's ends when he does. Has it come to this? Is desirability in a mate founded on how well you can take care of each other financially after the splendid years of youth and energy have gone? Come on, Jeanne, you've lost track of what is real, and economics is not the driving force for what matters.

What Is Real?

{March 3}

I AM ALSO losing track of where I left off.

Here's some imagery. Obviously there is still debris in my eye. Less and less. It needs to be cleaned up, and the macrophages (white blood cells) do it. The blood vessels need to dilate a little to let them through. Since November the debris has only thinned out. If they are attacking the Thing, creating more garbage, it does not show, there is no sensation from swelling or increased size, so whatever it is, it is not getting larger. Today I'm of a mind to let nature take its course.

Speaking of the left side of my face, I found a picture drawn by Mark White for a story I wrote called "The Wounded Healer," in *Shaman's Drum*, about twelve years ago. It was a woman's face, with a big tear spilling out of her left eye. Amazing little coincidence. Maybe I should go back and read what I've written before someone quotes me to me again.

Talked to my literary agent, Stephanie, today. She asked about the audience for this alleged book here. It's every single health consumer, and that's the truth. We have to get conscious.

The new health mandate for the year 2000 is "medical mistakes." Headlines. News releases. Target for our government. A couple of weeks ago, President Bill Clinton spoke of his commitment to review medical error and patient safety issues; Health and Human Services Secretary Donna Shalala made a personal commitment to improving the quality of health care, focusing on medical mistakes. Yesterday there

219

was a major story from Staten Island University Hospital: world-class surgeon has been operating wildly, even cutting on the wrong side of the brain of several patients. Another guy was fined for carving his initials on a woman's stomach while performing a cesarean. This is just the tip of the iceberg, folks. So I checked the Net. Surgical errors account for about 50 percent of all medical errors, according to a Harvard study published in the *New England Journal of Medicine*. Medicine is the third leading cause of death in the United States, right after heart disease and cancer. And we're not talking here about inappropriately prescribed treatments or medications; we're talking about those that are regarded as "standard of care."

I'm not saying my case represents a medical mistake. We won't know that until a pathologist looks at my eye after it is outside my body—which I hope will be never or a long time from now. But my case certainly represents medical confusion, at least my own.

Stephanie asks me whether I think people with other kinds of problems could relate to my experience.

"Of course. I don't think it matters too much whether it's your balls or your breasts or your eye. You are still in the same system, you are still faced with decisions, your life is still going down a significantly changed path, and one of great confusion." This very day a study about the highly positive effect of marijuana on brain cancer in rats makes the news. We're being bombarded with paradox. And last week there was something about the health-enhancing properties of chocolate for people with heart disease. And we know sex is good for everything. Sex, drugs, and chocolate—can't get much better than that. And here we all were, worrying about how to increase the fiber in our diets and whether we should walk fast, run, or what in order to keep fit.

———◇———

Back to the Tony thing. I wonder what he'd think if he knew his gorgeous one was fighting for her life. We are both a little worried about reopening a chapter that was never really finished. He does not, he says, want to regress to where he's been. He's "OK" now and wants to keep it that way. We have no future together, as best I can determine from my vantage point—married and not likely to change that status anytime in this lifetime, as far as I know.

He writes, "Years of dreaming of once again finding you have come to an end. Now what? I've spent my life loving the memories of loving you. I want to spend the remainder of my life loving those memories." I am touched by his sensitivity and awed at the responsibility we share in each other's lives.

Physicist John Stewart Bell said that once two protons have touched each other, their behavior continues to affect each other, no matter where they go in time or space. A theory with some credibility and a little research, if I remember quantum physics correctly.

Tony and I decided to send each other a series of short descriptions of significant events in our lives. Since he is a natural writer, I encouraged him to do this for himself, his nine grandchildren, and me. I'm wondering how to reciprocate and thinking maybe I could just send him chunks of this thing here that I'm writing. He'll probably cancel his subscription when he finds out about the true me, as Frank suggested.

Tony's first entry was a clear description of the moment we met—and he asked what I was thinking at the time. I don't recall, honestly. I just remember that we argued for the sake of arguing for a while, trying to keep some distance. He mentioned he did not like the way I looked from the rear after I came back from counseling at a summer camp. I'd gained some weight (up to 110), and my butt bounced. Wouldn't he just die if he knew that's what I remembered?

Regardless of whether I remembered, the moment was important to him: it was, he says, the basic theme of his life. "Good things happen to me as if someone is watching and protecting me."

Whatever this is all about, Tony certainly came into my life at the right time again. I was feeling fatally flawed as a woman, didn't know exactly why, and most of those issues were now overflowing the files in my mental file cabinet. I would need to do some cleaning soon.

I'm really getting all the unfinished business piled in front of me. What an opportunity. In self-defense I'm trying to think what else is out there that needs healing and get ready for whoever or whatever shows up.

Old Bones

{March 9}

THE CONVERSATIONS in our big adobe on the hill have been scant and redundant.

"How was your day?"

"Busy."

"What did you do?"

"Saw lots of patients."

"Where did you go?"

"Oh, the usual places."

Pause.

"How was your day?"

"Same old stuff—reading, writing, and talking on the phone."

"What do you want to do for dinner?"

End of dialogue, the long version, which I bet the birdkids, if we still had them, would have easily mastered by now. The reason I quit talking to Frank very much was a last-ditch effort to get him to talk to me about his secrets. Maybe this is a woman thing, but I'd tried everything else short of following him around all the time or hiring a detective. I do not know why he quit talking about his life or when. I must have made up things, "creative interpretations," to fill in the blanks.

Frank pecked me on the head with a good-bye kiss this morning, though, and called at noon. Maybe this will work out after all.

◇

Old bones with deliberate scratch marks are found all over the world, dating back to the beginning of time practically. This must have been how calendar records were kept, how menstrual cycles were tracked. These past few weeks have been so complicated, I could barely have made a scratch on a wall, or a bone, to mark the passage of time, much less have written in a journal.

Frank and I went to Hilton Head last week to do a conference for the National Institute for the Clinical Application of Behavioral Medicine. Long trip, intense conference, but the participants were bright and lively, the beach sweet, and the air soft. We had lunch with Stanley Krippner and Henry Dreher. Both are an answer to my recent prayers, as in, "Please, God, send me someone who knows immunology and someone who understands dreams."

Stanley looked at the symbols Frank had written during his dream night and interpreted them as announcements or heralds of healing. He seemed a little hesitant to make suggestions, but then Stan is not prone to imposing his own ideas. Both he and Henry believed that the "58" and "84" were good omens, since I am fifty-eight now and will probably live to be at least eighty-four. I agreed, it felt like that to me also.

Besides being a journalist, Henry is also a world-class repository of knowledge about the immune system. I later sent him my health history, and he carefully researched "my case."

Henry concluded that I might have had a delayed-type hypersensitivity (DTH) response, which could have caused the Event in the hotel in November. As per Elsa's ideas, he suggested that my imagery might best be focused on what was probably significant destruction of delicate structures. He pointed out, as did Mark Rennecker, how extremely reactive this class of tumor is to the immune system and gave me references to animal studies, including a mouse study in which fully 20 percent of the mice with transplanted ocular melanomas had a spontaneous remission.

Henry said, "It's the DTH that can potentially damage structures in the eye and therefore must be properly inhibited. But it is also DTH, I believe, that may in part be able to vanquish ocular melanoma. So it may be kind of a tightrope . . . some DTH but not too much may help to eliminate melanoma cells in the eye without destroying ocular structures."

He described other findings that suggest that the immune response in the eye is regulated by light and dark, via the effect on neuropeptides, the chemical messengers associated with the emotions as well as the immune system. "Intriguing, don't you think, that light and darkness may play a role in regulating our immune responses in the eye via mediators of the mind? What does that say about imagery, about light and shadow, about the balance that is life-sustaining? About the need to shift our state of mind, heart, environment to meet internal challenges to our physical integrity? Isn't it interesting that the eye is such a self-contained unit, and yet it can still be so influenced by light and dark and by the central nervous system? The eye is like one of those exclusive New York nightclubs where it's really hard to get past the doorman at the velvet ropes, but with the proper credentials or cachet, it's still possible."

Then he wrote, "I get the feeling that you somehow rode that razor's edge, sometimes guiding and sometimes witnessing an incendiary event in your own body, one that was fiery enough to burn out a tumor but not so explosive that it destroyed beyond function the delicate structures in the anterior chamber of your eye."

Well, no wonder I had been seeking dark places, trying to sleep, keeping my eyes closed.

I bought a suitcase full of the kind of exquisite summer clothes you only find at high-end stores in classy resort hotels: a three-piece cream stretchy lace outfit with long skirt and jacket; a slinky long black dress with a black lace top; light blue slacks, matching sweater, and a jacket made of fantasy cloth. Great stuff. I have this theory that the outfits I buy determine in advance my future, and there is something to this—perhaps it is not a determining factor but a certain intuition or inner knowing of what's ahead, like when you pick up the telephone before it rings or use a dowsing rod to find water. People do this all the time. Think I'll go shopping after I finish writing today to see what I buy.

I want to point out one more time that I'm buying things for the coming season—that is, the future—which is a good sign. These clothes were drop-dead gorgeous, and they eventually went to an exotic, warm place where I had no idea I would be going.

When Frank and I returned home, we spent two days tidying up business, running like squirrels in a wheel, and then another bomb dropped. Ed Tyska blew his head off with a gun. Not possible, I think. Not Ed. His lifestyle was so pristine. How could he even touch a gun? He was as beautiful as he was kind—never a silver hair out of place in his pompadour; soft, glowing skin; his sixty-six years remarkably unmarred by time. The imagery of what happened—Ed splattered over the kitchen—made me violently ill, and I threw up all one afternoon. When a friend called Frank to tell him, she said, "and a few days before he was just saying how he loved Jeannie so much." Ed is one of the seventeen people in the world who still refer to me as Jeannie. He'd called me several times over the past few months, always reminding me that "you are not your body."

Ed knew as much medicine as Andy Weil and Deepak Chopra, but he never had the charisma for show business. He unstintingly did service with the Unity Church in Dallas for as long as I'd known him. We had multiple relationships: he was the only physician I trusted with my health when I lived in Dallas, he was a colleague, and he was a student in many of my programs, including the year-long imagery training program. His death, violent though it was, freed his restless spirit to do healing work from another dimension. I will ask him to make a house call once he gets settled.

And, by the way, I am thoroughly, absolutely, completely disgusted with the eye. It may have gotten better last week and let in more light, but who would know because I hid my face from the world mourning Ed? When the light shifts, I feel seasick and disoriented. I have to squint to walk. I don't try to drive. I've given up being the Olympic Shopping Champion of the World. Unfamiliar, large stores are impossible terrain because they are too highly textured and usually too dark to navigate without getting confused.

I finished the mistletoe series, which meant six days of relatively high doses. I cooked—not cold fire this time but hot flashes. I woke up early, bathed in sweat. I want to poke my own eye out. I'm so sick of it. The physical appearance continues to get better—others say. The iris is mostly green. It is not much more bloodshot than the other eye—and what the hell do you expect from the other one, since I've been writing all day again and need a cane to stand up from the computer? The yellow crap in the anterior chamber is still there, and when viewed in the sunlight, I look just plain weird. Fleur said the Eye didn't look bad; it simply looked as if it were taking a little vacation.

Frank says I look exotic—but he lies a lot, probably to make me feel better. The yellow sea in the middle is still thinning, and I can see pinpoints of black, which must mean the pupil shows in tiny places. My cornea is clear and seems to be intact. I still take the enzymes from Germany. Sometimes I take liver-support things, too, like SAMe and milk thistle.

I had one profound message from wherever these things come from. Dreams. Meditations. It was, "Get rid of the fish." The fish have been the theme of the white blood cells. The fish came in first to dismantle the DNA. We bought a big white coy and called him the macrophage. I dreamed the fish had killed other fish and then died. Now something says to get rid of the fish.

To me, getting rid of the fish meant, "Stop the inflammation." It could mean to stop the mistletoe and other immune stimulators. It does feel like systemic stimulation with no target. It could mean the immune system has got out of hand—as in autoimmunity—and needs a signal to quit. It could also mean that the dead fish have left debris and that needs to be cleansed. My intuition says to go into cleansing and detoxification mode and forget the stimulation for now. Carl has been thinking and talking to people, and he gets the same hit from his own inner wisdom. He's sending me a case of magnetized water from Japan, which has some research suggesting it enters the forbidden zone of the ocular system. Of course, I'll give it a shot. I need something to wash out the fish parts.

Jean Bolen called and remarked that Someone has given me a post-graduate course in life. But what do I do after I graduate? I threw an *I Ching* to look for an answer. I didn't like the first *I Ching* I threw, so I threw another and another until I got Youthful Folly, which means you've asked the same question too damn many times. The morass of information, before Youthful Folly, didn't contain particularly good news. What the *I Ching* said was to keep focused on teaching and not expect too much too soon. Springs don't fill up instantly: there is a trickle and then a flow. And no, I am not out of danger, and I must not forgot that. It said that if you ignore danger, you get creamed, or something of that nature.

My body wisdom is only *really* clear on what not to do right now: don't let the eye get tossed on the slag heap.

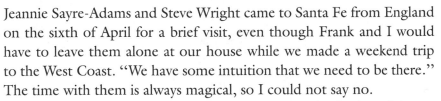

Jeannie Sayre-Adams and Steve Wright came to Santa Fe from England on the sixth of April for a brief visit, even though Frank and I would have to leave them alone at our house while we made a weekend trip to the West Coast. "We have some intuition that we need to be there." The time with them is always magical, so I could not say no.

The first day they were in Santa Fe, we went to the healing shrine at Chimayó and came home with dirt from a hole in a side chapel and several bottles of holy water from the fountain. The church is always filled with the intoxicating smell and light of hundreds of candles offered as prayers and the sounds of weeping and gratitude. The second day of their visit, April 7, Frank and I left before breakfast for San Francisco.

Birthday

{April 7}

TODAY, THE DAY BEFORE my birthday, I did my last-minute shopping in the Denver International Airport mall, which is one of the finer shopping areas around—or maybe that's just my personal illusion because I don't get out much anymore. I bought a dress by a favorite Italian designer. One of a kind, made of blue lace, fairylike, and hand-dyed in vats in a family business in southern Italy. There are not many of these outfits around because the family designs and produces when and what it pleases. My eagle couture eye spotted them at a great distance. As the outfit was being thrown into a bag, I realized it cost my entire honorarium for the talk. What the hell. Bury me in it.

Following our arrival in California, Frank and I celebrated my upcoming birthday by having dinner at our favorite seafood restaurant in Ghirardelli Square. Although the restaurants and bars have changed names over the years, we shared many memorable occasions on these premises overlooking the most famous bridge in the world and the mists of San Francisco Bay. Once we stayed until the wee hours at the Pacific Bar and Grill, which is no longer there, and sketched our theory about life and the hereafter on a single napkin. I still have it. The napkin provided the material for at least one book and conversation for years afterward.

This evening, though, I was weepy and almost too tired to eat.

"Frank," I said, "things are not going well for us. My fondest desire is that we both find happiness and fulfillment, and that we do it gently, gracefully, and without hurting each other." Tears drizzled down my cheeks, and I wiped them away with a napkin, managing to smear crab cake on my face in the process.

This conversation came on the heels of a medium-big fight between Frank and me right before Jeannie and Steve had arrived. I had been on one of my economizing jags, which come with fatigue, and images of the Bag Lady archetype were dogging my thoughts. I brought up the touchy issue of finances. The specter of not being able to keep up my pace and income made me wild, and we had no other game plan in sight to support our future.

Economics had become the current battleground for our personal dynamics, but it was just a symptom of long-standing, deeply buried turbulence. With few exceptions psychologists don't earn much, and many academics live in genteel poverty, so we are not talking large sums here.

After my comments Frank ran downstairs, and I followed like a stalker. "Please look at me while we talk," I said, after cornering him at his desk.

"No, that is one thing I never will have to do again. Look at you. And I don't have to answer your questions. My business is my business, and yours is yours. Boundaries have always been a problem for you." I'm filing this one away, too, in the very top drawer of the mental file cabinet, the one labeled "Mysteries." The next morning I wrote Frank a note saying that the problem was not finances at all but that I did not feel cared for.

On the eve of my birthday, at the fish restaurant, Frank gave me a piece of turquoise-colored stone I had admired weeks earlier in the glass case of a local jewelry store. It is circled by silver and will slip over a chain. It is beautiful, and like all things in nature, it is made more beautiful by its imperfections. I love it. Frank appreciated and designed unique jewelry, and I have a treasure chest full of his gifts. He made me a birthday card on his computer: "We have had a year of challenges, and we will likely have more. We can overcome anything. Remember, you will always be my bride." Lovely. I drop the discussion of going our separate ways. I really am just tired, that's all.

April 8 was the longest day in history. I completely forgot the eye, except when I had to negotiate the steps onto a stage in an auditorium at the University of San Francisco Medical School.

We had spent the night in a hotel above the corner where more pedestrians and bicyclists are killed on the crosswalk than any other place in San Francisco. Three were felled before morning. The noise was amazing—unnatural sounds that I didn't know existed. Four hours of sleep.

The next morning I spoke to a group of the most interested, kind, organized, and bright-eyed medical students I have ever seen. Hundreds of them. Alternative therapy is not a bizarre interest or a hobby but appears deeply ingrained in their belief systems. Medicine may be changing before our very eyes. The lecture was at some ungodly hour like 8:00 A.M. I did a decent job in my Denver International Airport swooping, pale blue lace ensemble. You can wear these costumes on the West Coast. Friends were in the audience and obviously glad to see me alive, and I was flattered that they had come to hear me rant and rave one more time.

Just to give a picture of the day: After the lecture Frank picked me up on a windy corner, and we drove down the coast to an engagement party for Judy's daughter, Kerri, held at Pajaro Dunes in her father's exquisite home-to-die for on the beach. This willowy young woman, a member of the "lost generation," had found herself. She is a survivor, successful, and just plain nice.

Then we left to go find my son, Chase, in the northern California mountains, and I steeled myself for the contrast. He was in his hovel, naked, covered with bug bites, and when he emerged into the sun, his pupils were pinpricks. He was bathed in sweat and covered with dog hair. When I saw him, I wanted to crawl into a rabbit hole and never come out. Frank greeted him, and we made a deal for brunch the next day. It was nearly Chase's birthday also.

After we left, I was silent and sick on the winding road down to Big Sur, where my daughter lived in one room, with outdoor bath facilities, no heat, and a not very wonderful picture of me hanging above the bed like an icon. She is joyous, hospitable, and not at all unhappy. She is still partly paralyzed, and her sight is challenged, as they say, but she is as fine as she ever gets.

We took her down the coast to Jerry Schiff's place on Pfeiffer Ridge, where we would be spending the night in his newly built guesthouse, perched on the edge of the world. Only twenty-six families lived on the ridge when Frank and I were there, and four of us were born on April 8, which defies some kind of odds. Many others were Aries, including Frank. What this means is up for grabs, and it may mean nothing at all. Ram Ridge, it was called, and we always had a birthday party at Jerry's place. It was typical Big Sur: some celebrations may have lasted a couple of days. Once you got to a party way up on the ridge, it was tempting not to go home until you got good and ready or had to leave for work.

Of the original April 8 group, only Jerry was left on the ridge now; the others had died or moved away. Returning on our mutual birthday felt important this year of my presumed demise. Jerry had champagne on ice, birthday cake, and plans for dinner. I lasted just long enough to eat an appetizer, confirming, I suppose, my mortal illness and not how busy I had been since 6:00 o'clock that morning.

On Sunday we went back to Chase's. He had cleaned up and was a shadow of his delicately beautiful self—strawberry hair (which came from who knows where) and tiger eyes (also source unknown), but with pinprick pupils still. While we were waiting in line for brunch in a nearby village, he and I darted out to a store and bought him a pair of shoes, engineered for running, hiking, or just many hours afoot. His neighbor had told me that Chase was "afoot" most of the time, so he was obviously walking off his troubling inner world. As far as I could tell, the old shoes accounted for at least half the nasty smells that permeated the air between Chase and me, but he insisted on taking them home in a box nevertheless.

Chase and Frank carried on their FBI and CIA discussions at lunch, and I wanted to put my fist in my mouth to stifle screams. Instead, I did the decent thing and dissociated, staring into space or down at my cupped hands.

Since I had business in San Francisco the next day, we drove up the coast, Frank dropped me off at Mo's, then he went back to Santa Fe. That night Judy and Mo took me to one of our dinners that made us thankful to be together for these significant occasions and to have taste buds. We have been known to dig into the lamb with both hands and throw the bones in the hearth. I always justify this to myself by remembering the story of Saint Teresa of Ávila (there I go again, trying to compare us to saints, but Teresa was lively), who was caught devouring a partridge with both hands in the kitchen late one night. "When I pray, I pray; when I eat partridge, I eat partridge." Actually, this is pretty Zen. Pay attention. Stay awake.

The girlfriends have decided that I have not been taking care of myself, and I don't, except for a loud outfit now and then. I buy hairbrushes with the groceries and other necessities at the discount stores. For my birthday they gave me my first and only pair of black lace panties from a French designer, which must have cost more than the dinner itself. "Miss Jeanne, you need to fix yourself up a little," said Judy.

"But these things don't have a cotton crotch."

"Don't worry about it."

Twilight Zone

{April 11}

IN THE MEANTIME Jeannie and Steve had a rough stay in our house. Steve, hypersensitive to nuances of energy that are beyond perception to most of us, had dream battles every single night. He felt that something terrible had happened on the property and in the house; that I really needed protection, and the home and grounds needed cleansing.

"Something here endangers Jeanne's life," Steve said, and Frank agreed but said he had not gotten around to doing anything about it. Steve was shocked at his response. When I got home, I found a small medicine wheel made of rose quartz on the front of the property, built where Steve felt the most disturbance. The critters scatter the rocks every night, but I have tried to keep it intact. After leaving Santa Fe, Jeannie and Steve took the indirect route back to England through San Francisco and expressed their fears to Judy. "What can we do to help her?" they asked. "We do not feel that she is safe."

Judy suggested they make every effort to find a way to help, because they were not alone in their concerns.

After returning home, I felt like a piece of dog doo-doo and took to my bed. I now have this theory that the longer you spend stifling your screams, the longer it takes to recover. Frank looked in on me every few hours when he was home. He wrote and told people that he thought my medical condition had worsened significantly and he was waiting and watching, and making plans to move to Texas . . . "if." Or more dismally "when," which I thought was slightly pessimistic.

233

Shit. I had a case of the vapors, darling. Every decent woman in the nineteenth century knew about vapors. Later they started calling it a nervous breakdown. I am sure Frank thought it was organ failure.

One night he bolted up off the couch and said, "I need to call Carl right away." He left a message for Carl in such a strange voice that Carl hardly recognized it. Carl called me back on my line and said, "What's going on sweetheart? Pancho [which is what he calls Frank] says he thinks you are going downhill fast. But that isn't why he called me. I don't know why he called, actually."

"I'm in hell again. Just saw my son."

"Well, no wonder you took to your bed."

After returning home to the space vacated by Jeannie and Steve, I had three days in which to have my nervous breakdown, and then family company came, so I had to straighten up and get with the program. My niece Tami, her husband, Dan, and her mom, JoLynn (who remains my sister-in-law regardless of whether she's married to my brother), as well as Baby Nolan graced our home with their lively presences.

On the second night of their visit, Tami let out a bloodcurdling scream and came running out of the hall in the guest wing. "Please hold my hand." I turned the lights on, and her face was white and her eyes huge. I held her hand and led her down the stairs.

"For crying out loud, Tami, what is going on?"

She stammered, "Something was there, like death, a déjà vu, my dead grandmother—no, I don't know what it was. Something terrible." She trembled all evening and never forgot it. Tami is a grounded, intelligent young woman, with no forays, that I am aware of, into the supernatural. What she was trying to describe was a compilation of every weird experience she had ever had. She is sensitive but not a hysteric. She had absolutely no idea what she saw. This was the hall near the kitchen where the dogs had refused to walk. It was also near where Jeannie and Steve had been sleeping nights earlier, when Steve had been battling the forces of darkness. It is absolutely beautiful, and the rooms have a view of the mountain and native piñons and junipers. At night the stars look like something out of a Disneyland production, and in the moonlight the animals put on quite a show, with rabbits hopping and coyotes yowling and a pair of owls flying around the property. We are not talking ugly here or unnatural; but we are talking strange.

Healing Island

{April 25}

BY THE LAST WEEK in April, company was gone, I was rested, and I packed my Hilton Head finery into my suitcase to go to the *Alternative Therapies* conference in Kona, Hawaii. Since I was on sabbatical from the journal and not the lead dog this year—only introducing speakers and doing a couple of sessions—my accommodations were not the executive suites to which I had been accustomed. In fact, I was in an airless room behind a berm. No stretch limo met me. Was this going to be fun or what? It was fun. A single yoga session on the beach at sunrise and I went, plunk, back into my body from wherever I had wandered.

The perfumed air and volcanic beaches, among other things, are what entitle this place to call itself the healing island. Elders from all the other islands came here periodically for teaching and initiation. This year I decided to get a suntan. Who cared? It would make me look and feel better. Anyway, life might be shorter than I had previously anticipated, and I might not need to worry so much about getting basal cell carcinoma when I'm eighty. Seemed like such a small problem in the overall scheme of things.

In Kona I felt as though I had come to some level place where the worst was behind me.

I had a quick lunch with Jim Gordon and Susan Lord, the physicians who had invited me to travel to the Balkans—and incidentally changed my life. Susan was leading a workshop on how to embark on the clinical practice of alternative medicine, and Jim was taking a few precious days off to sleep, bodysurf, and hang out. As usual, our conversations were brilliant and compelling, if I do say so myself. We talked about transformations of life in all their manifestations. Susan said, "You are the perfect example of energy transformation. You transformed a terrible tumor, a piece of physical matter, into energy!" She was right, I did have energy, more than I could ever remember having, and it was only in the past few days that I'd come to realize that I was well rid of whatever dark and malevolent force had taken up residence in my life.

Back in September, when Michael Harner had connected with the spirits that speak to him, they said I had more work to do. I had no idea then that the healing island of Hawaii would be the location for my destined work.

———⟡———

When I returned home to Santa Fe three days later, everything had changed. I tried to drive into the three-car garage, which is bigger than most houses in the United States, and couldn't park without running into or over some kind of trash. My senses were assaulted by screwdrivers, wires, dirty pillows, a tractor covered with God knows what, a broken statue of our Lady of Guadelupe, a woodpile gone awry, old mail, boxes of journals, junk from nearby construction sites, not to mention the dirt on the floor. Everything was tumbling over everything else. Old rubbish, stained pieces of foam rubber, and frayed blankets had been pulled out of the trash and thrown on the floor. Doggie-damaged door screens were propped randomly against the wall awaiting repair. Nests were everywhere, and the smell of rodents was overpowering.

Had this just happened? No, of course not. I must have seen it before, upped my tolerance level, and then blocked it out. Once a month or so, I had feebly shoved a push broom around to keep the New Mexico dirt at bay and picked up the papers and food wrappers that littered the floor around the trash can. There was nothing more I could do about it. It was too much.

This was not about a dirty garage. I really didn't give a rat's ass about dirty garages. This was a shock of reentry to something I did not fully remember—a metaphor, in case I'm not making my point clear.

When I got into the house, it was as if the furniture had been moved around, but it was all in its same old places. The most startling disarray was more intangible: it was psychic, energetic. It wasn't as though something was missing but rather as if something had been added.

The once-a-week housekeeper had been avoiding doing anything in some rooms where paper and other flotsam and jetsam of an organic and inorganic nature were multiplying; she had simply been doing a quick sweep-out of the center of the floor. How long had this been going on—this mess and the whirlwind of something that could not be named blowing through these beautiful spaces?

Fire in the Mountain

{May 6}

THE WEEK AFTER HAWAII I was totally and deliciously well—better than well, feeling *good*. I dressed in long skirts, embroidered blouses, and always one of my many hats—knockoffs from the Victorian or Edwardian era. Suitably gowned, I went to the health food store, the dry cleaner's, and ran all those errands that had been neglected during the Bad Dream. In Santa Fe everyone looks as if he or she had just come from central casting, even at the grocery store, which is what makes it a better place to live than Newark.

I spent hours in an absolute, unmitigated trance in the nurseries and greenhouses. It was time to get the gardens planted, and what indescribable joy! Tomatoes had already been set out in blue plastic water wells, which are really solar collectors, to make sure they would ripen before the frost. Santa Fe has a growing season of about 110 days, so you have to be quick on your feet and time your plantings carefully after the last freeze. Now was the season to plant red and yellow and purple and green lettuces, yellow and orange nasturtiums amid the cucumbers and marigolds. Zinnias. Berries and grapes. Peas and green beans. A special plot for corn and the ancient beans that were found in the Anasazi dwellings. My veggie and cut-flower garden is designed like an Italian herb garden, with walkways, four major beds, and a small, square planting in the center. This summer white roses, planted the year before, would climb over the wooden coyote fence that keeps the rabbits out of the salad. Carol, my spiritual gardener, came in and planted seeds for Cinderella pumpkins, so orange they glow in the dark, and squashes that grow, no kidding, to two feet long.

A clay angel with wings bigger than she was sat with her hand under her chin on the edge of one of the beds. Tibetan chimes rang from the center tripod, and on each clanger we had tied a paper with a prayer.

Springtime in the garden is a tribute to life. I was alive! Pheromones were sparkling off my body like gold dust; with the music and gardens and sunlight and everything, I was so sensuous, I did not think it would be a good idea to be in a crowd in my condition. Everyone would know how I was feeling, heads would turn, and I would surely become the Pied Piper, with men following me home.

"Frank, it would be so wonderful to have a weekend of wild love-making. I want to do that."

"So do I," he said.

A shadow crossed my mind, and it was one of those times when you don't know whether it is a memory or a fragment from an old, forgotten dream or whether a veil between the worlds has lifted for an instant. Or maybe it was nothing, perhaps just the wind. In any event, I knew in that moment that I would never be the initiatrix for the most intimate of all engagements with him again, ever, in this life or any life to come.

After lunch on Saturday, Frank told me he had scheduled sessions at the homes of patients both that afternoon and the next. I asked him why he would do that on a weekend, during our play time.

"It's a window of time."

"What do you mean, 'a window of time'?"

"Just what I said, a window."

"What is a 'window'?"

"Just that. What I said. A window."

Obviously we were not going to spend an intimate weekend.

On Sunday afternoon, when he left with a camera and a tripod sticking out from under his arm to videotape a patient doing exercises in her studio, I knew that this would not be a regular patient session and that he would be gone long enough for me to do some thinking. The time had well nigh come to clean out the drawers of the mental file cabinet. Mind you, it was not because I was sick but because I was well; not because I was dying but because I wanted to stay alive at whatever cost.

After he left, I went out into the garden and began scraping, pounding, digging, mulching, and praying about what I must do regarding my work in this lifetime that was yet undone. I'm not sure to whom I was praying, but it was something like, "Please, God, send me a sign."

My dream of two summers ago returned: I was struck as if by a fiery bolt while mulching my garden by the gate and woke with a start with the sun in my face. Without a millisecond of thought, I threw down the trowel, ran up the road, dashed up the stairs into the house, and yanked open a drawer in a seldom-used wicker desk in the back room. The contents flew across the floor—coins, combs, pens, cards, and the scraps of paper that I had smushed into wads last November right before the eye incinerated. As with the house and garage, it seemed like someone had rearranged things—or had I just not been paying attention?

With beads of moisture forming on my face and prickles on my arms, I sorted through all that stuff—and I found it. There had been clues all along. I had had hunches, but a scientist needs hard data. It's not appropriate for me to go into the sordid details here, but suffice to say that Frank was not the man I thought he was. Dark secrets unraveled. On this, my very brightest, healthiest day in years, lightning struck stone and blasted the illusion to dust.

At this very same hour, despite the imminent danger of high winds and drought conditions, a "controlled burn" was started near Los Alamos. Trees, brush, mercury, plutonium, and whatever else they won't admit began to smolder and then blaze, and houses exploded. A toxic cloud spread for hundreds of miles or maybe forever. From my bedroom window, I could see sparking flares of red in the distance.

The microcosm of my small and insignificant life was here, reflected in this tragedy, which continued throughout the summer. The planet's most advanced technologists had not cleaned up their wastes. Here was the birthplace of the creations of legendary and brilliant minds, not just for the purposes of defense but for medicine and energy and technology that took us into the space age. What had been stored underground and ignored for so long had now erupted and was poisoning the skies.

A forest fire this was not, and it was out of control. I knew forest fires well after Big Sur—how they looked and smelled, how to calculate danger as ash rained on the roof and helicopters whirred incessantly overhead while we watched for flames to leap a ridge, being prepared to throw the living creatures and valuables into the car and take an escape route. Fire is a natural means of purging and cleansing and ensures new growth in the springtime; we all knew that and respected the dangers. This, I repeat, was not a natural fire, and no amount of water or trenching or fire retardant would halt its relentless march.

No mediation was possible; there was no longer a healing solution for either Los Alamos or us. It was not the last act—the small fire that ignited the dry brush—that caused the damage; it was the years of neglect, the secret cover-ups, ignorance, superficial but glamorous success, pretense. And finally, in the last analysis, it was the inability to rectify, with truth-telling and forgiveness, what had been too long festering underground.

Surgery

{May 9}

I FLED TO A SANCTUARY in the mountains for five days, climbed the rocks, sat in a limestone cave, wrote, prayed as best I could, and tried to figure things out. Fleur Green, who would be my therapist if she were not my friend, insisted on meeting me somewhere for dinner almost every night. She held on to me so I did not do a half gainer and flip out of time and space. She and the other local girlfriends, Barbie Dossey and Sandy Ingerman, did the loving equivalent of sitting me down and throwing cold water in my face to try to bring me out of shock. The telephone rang often, and the massive support network rallied once again.

Tony, the man whom I had not seen in about half a century, connected with me daily, not to encourage me to do one thing or another but to remind me that I was a good woman, whatever happened. His support was inestimable. For the second time he saved my life. Much earlier he had assured me that I was among the most beautiful and desirable of God's creations, and I believed him. The impression of my own self-worth was a cushion that buoyed me through most of my life. Now Tony had come back into my life to help me remember that I was of value, just when I most needed to hear it again. He is a medicine man without a tribe, and his medicine is unfailing kindness.

In the time of retreat on the mountain, I was absentmindedly aware only that something was happening to the eye. No pain or swelling, but white streaks were forming across the iris, like kite strings from the anterior chamber.

Over the five days, the sky got whiter and turned to gauze. And then black. Where I was staying, two older people checked out early, saying they couldn't breathe. I could still breathe, but the in-breath tasted like metal, and it wasn't too long before I felt like a piece of aluminum. I had to go home soon; the cloud was drifting across the highway. As I pulled out onto the road, a raven died and fell from the sky.

———◇———

On our twenty-third anniversary, the fifteenth of May, I filed for divorce. I spent the day preparing an album of our life together. On the front page I placed the gold medallion, a double circle with a cross, that Frank had made for me and placed on my neck the afternoon we were married in a field of wildflowers. I had worn it for most of our time together. It had symbolized so much for us: the joining of the masculine and feminine, the holy and enduring connection, the blessings and challenges that can only be encountered when hearts are dedicated. We had written stories and poetry about the symbolic meaning; it was of the ancient magi, Carl Jung knew it well, it had been cherished by many lovers and esoteric philosophers. It was no longer fitting that it should be mine.

The album contained pictures of our adventures, stunning venues, spectacular homes in paradise, our children as they grew, our noteworthy colleagues; but mostly the pictures were of us—always close, touching, playing, and usually in costumes. We were, so many said, simply beautiful together. My poetry was splattered through the book, and the last page showed a prince and princess kissing good-bye. "The End of the Dream." Frank perused the book and set it down beside his plate. "Wonderful," he said, and did not look at it again.

———◇———

Frank had left quickly that day, with no questions asked, no faltering, no requests for mediation. For another week, or maybe it was two or three, I watched the flames, the smoke, and the embers; prepared to drive to California if it got any worse. I answered calls, did the work that I have done for so long I can do it in my sleep, scheduled and rescheduled my life.

I did not leave Frank's side of the bed, except to care for the pups and the gardens and the fish. The atmosphere of the home and land-scape of the grounds were surreal and acted in stewardship for my safety during the fugue.

Twice, out of incredible loneliness and sorrow, I recanted my decision for separation and suggested we consider a different, ordinary, plain life. A bait shop in Hawaii, a retreat in Costa Rica. Go someplace where no one knew who we were. We had the resources to begin another life together, but it must be new and far away. Or he could go on retreat, take a year or more off, partake of solitude and spiritual counsel.

Unbeknownst to me during my bargaining to be together at whatever cost, within hours after signing the interim agreement in May, Frank had arranged to have the woman in California who answered telephones for a living join him as a partner for what he considered his true destiny as an average man. Divorced now, she sold her house and moved her furniture to Dallas before summer's end. Their condo is conventional and in an average neighborhood. She stays home all day to care for Frank's needs.

I have no idea how Frank weathered the hellfires of the divorce, but he did not do it alone. I can only assume he has a comfortable home close to his family and culture and is finally content. He left his professional work in psychology and alternative and complementary medicine as quickly as he did the state of New Mexico and now works in the corporate world, he says, doing something with computer software. More than that I do not know.

I had amputated my soul mate in order to survive, and now I wasn't sure I would survive such serious surgery. Two rough diamonds, we had polished each other's edges until we had reached a molten core. We were both in grave danger of loss of soul, if indeed that had not already occurred. I live in the mystery of how this could have happened with the one person I loved more than my life. Except it did, and it happened when I began to fall in love with myself again. Whatever work I had left to do, it must be done alone for now.

The grief was indescribable; the air around me was leaden and so very still that nothing but the patterns of the sky seemed to move. I was incredulous that my life had been spared for this. Maybe there was no larger story after all. I was in a big house with two dogs, major expenses, monumental work commitments, an uncertain future, maybe dying, absolutely more alone than I had ever been in my life, and had a very dirty garage. So what good were all the healing ceremonies, the positive intentions, the thousands of prayers made on my behalf, my own hard work to change my life and invite my vision to return? Had they brought me to this, the darkest place of grief? Death would have been easier.

The fires of Los Alamos eventually died down at the end of August, but the wastes burned for months and may be burning still.

Psyche's Challenges

THERE WAS A LARGER STORY being played out, and I knew well what it was. I had been touched by something far greater than ordinary human experience, and the myth of Psyche was a prescription for how to survive the "divine touching" (Robert Johnson's phrase from his exquisite rendition of the myth in *She*.) These old myths feel like real landscapes, inhabited by living people, the archetypes. They teach, enable humanity to evolve, and work on us until we become awake and conscious. Their stories live in our bones. Knowing the bigger picture helps us get through dry spells and dark nights, if only barely. Psyche had been doing a number on me in this regard for some time.

Psyche, a mortal woman, was in love with the god Eros, who gave her everything she wished in paradise. He came to her only in the darkness, though, and forbade her to inquire about any of his ways. Her sisters finally convinced her to take a lamp to her bed and shine it to see his face. The sleeping Eros was awakened when a drop of oil from the lamp fell on his right shoulder. Angry that Psyche had disobeyed him and fearful that she would see his true nature, he fled.

Four years ago Frank and I had a few therapy sessions with a male Jungian analyst who had studied Psyche. He maintained that girlfriends were always suspect, since Psyche was provoked into this intrusive act by her jealous sisters, and she paid dearly. An interesting interpretation, to say the least, and I wonder how common it is. It was the sisterhood that had collectively hinted (with the exception of Mo, who never beats around the bush about anything) that I should shine a light on my conjugal relationship and that it was not what I believed it to be.

For me relationship was spiritual practice. I did not expect perfection but rather challenge, and I had no illusions about Frank's being the God of love and my being a mortal woman who passed as a goddess with a cult following either. I had always longed to see his true nature, and, as with Psyche, it was kept secret.

When Psyche realized that Eros was lost to her, she tried to drown herself. Death, of course, is easier than living with such loss, and in these archetypal stories, you usually have a choice: collapse and die, or live and learn something. Psyche saved herself and asked Aphrodite what she should do to find her own godlike nature and happiness at last. She was assigned the four famous and nearly impossible tasks required of the mature feminine, each one building upon the others into a terrible crescendo, and then and only then could love return and Psyche give birth to Pleasure.

According to my singular interpretation, I'd been working my way through Psyche's assignments for some time. The first of her tasks was to sort an impossible variety of seeds, which I interpret as what I've been doing with my research and day jobs, not to mention my personal life. I'm trying to bring order out of chaos, map the unknown, and figure things out—to my satisfaction, at least. It makes me happy to use my linear mind to make categories and taxonomies out of image and prayer, love and intuition, and other worlds not visible to the naked eye. Psyche got a little help in the night from a small army of ants who organized the seeds, and maybe this is what happens to me with my dreams. The talent for analyzing and organizing and for orderly thought encroaches on the skills associated with the masculine, and as a woman in a world of men for all of my thirty professional years, it has rewarded me well.

The second task was to obtain a strand of golden fleece—another guy-type thing. The fleece is hair from a ferocious ram and must be taken with cunning or you get battered to death. The reeds in the river whispered to Psyche to collect strands left on the fences and do it at dusk so the rams would not see her. Gotcha. The golden fleece was the hero's booty, and you can get it without a power struggle. I never understood power struggles much anyway.

The third assignment was to drink a goblet of water from the River Styx. The river flowed in a circular course, from the mountains into the earth and back again, and the banks were guarded by monsters. Psyche could not approach the river herself and survive, so she commissioned an eagle with panoramic vision to carry the goblet for her and get the water. Eagles had appeared often enough recently for me to trust that they would bring me what I needed from the eternal river and that I did not have to do it all myself.

However, it is the fourth and final task that no one in his or her right mind would volunteer for, and I do not pretend to understand it fully. I am in the midst of dealing with this challenge and do not yet know how it will turn out. Psyche is instructed by Aphrodite to go to the Underworld and get a cask of beauty lotion or potion from Persephone. Persephone had been tricked into the nether regions by her attraction to the beautiful Narcissus, who was in love only with himself. Psyche is given tools for her journey—coins and barley bread. She has to cross the River Styx at night and pay the ferryman and quiet the barking dog. So far, I've been there, done that.

A drowning man reaches up from the water, and she must pass him by. A crippled donkey driver drops his wood and asks for help, and he, too, must be ignored or Psyche will not be able to find her way through this awful assignment. She has to bypass three women who are the Weavers of Fate and resist the temptation to join them. Finally she makes it to the Underworld and gets the beauty potion. The coast is clear. She travels back the same way she came and paradoxically decides to open the box or bottle or whatever it is instead of saving it for Aphrodite. Turns out it's not a beauty potion but a vapor of death. Psyche swoons. Eros gets wind that she is dying and intercedes with Aphrodite on her behalf. Psyche turns into a real live goddess and gives birth to a daughter, Pleasure.

With each challenge Psyche considers that drowning herself would be easier, especially (or maybe I'm projecting) when called upon to avoid the wounded men. As the story goes, a woman can only legitimately refuse to give compassionate assistance and pass through this task of individuation if she has already given fully of herself at some previous time. To continue to exhibit unbridled kindness, though, will diminish her capacity for loving others and living. Bypassing the Fates and resisting the opportunity to seize control over other people's lives is especially difficult when it comes to your children who are in trouble.

They are not my children, though, but children of life, and they—as well as the needy men—have their own contracts with Fate. I'm wrestling with all this, but at least Psyche has made me conscious of the tasks at hand.

I have not yet retrieved the cask of beauty secrets from the Underworld, returned, had a near-death experience, been rescued by a lover, or given birth to joy. I figure this is what my future holds, if everything goes according to plan.

Epilogue

{December 23, 2000}

ELEVEN MONTHS AGO TODAY, I began writing this journal to help me understand my metaphoric life and, if possible, to save my life. I had no idea how or when this epilogue would be written or where I would be. This week the wheel that began turning several years ago has come full circle, and I am ready to begin a new life.

I am in Big Sur, California, staying in a rustic cabin in the valley, under giant redwoods. I've come home, not only because this is the beautiful area where I lived longer than anyplace in my transient life but also because it is where I can be with my children. My daughter, Lee Ann, is living with a fine man who adores her, across the street from my cabin. Chase drove down. He is not himself, but he did show up.

We will spend Christmas Eve together for the first time in perhaps eight years, and my dread of the holidays has evaporated into gratitude. I never thought I, or they, would live long enough for us to be together again under the same roof.

We have already opened presents from my mother. She sent me a negligee—a leopard-spotted and black-lace affair. I can't imagine her even entering stores where such things are sold—which, if I remember correctly, are next to theaters that feature X-rated films. My son was appalled; my daughter, delighted. When I thanked Mom for it, she said, "Well, it is something to get you started. You need to find a man at least ten years younger than you. If they get much older, they start thinking old." Mom is planning my life again, but now it sounds OK to me.

I tried to have a couple of little talks with the kids, asking them to forgive me for not having paid enough attention to their needs, but each time both of them stopped me in midsentence and thanked me for their upbringing, because they said it gave them their strength and character. I finally shut up and sipped on the great French Chateneauf du Pape that Chase had brought for lunch.

This week I returned from the annual vacation at Kona Village on the Big Island; only this time I was alone with the girlfriends, if ever that can be termed alone. And this time it was not just a vacation but the beginnings of a relocation.

Last summer—in the days when I was most anxious, paralyzed with grief, still not stirring from Frank's side of the bed—I called a man whom I call a "spiritual" real estate agent, and told him I had to sell the house, rent it, do something.

He replied, "I can hear in your voice that you're in no condition to make such decisions right now. Why don't you try to take some quiet time out, pray or meditate if you can, but try to still your mind a little. Then call me back."

Very appropriate advice; even the real estate people were looking out for my best interests.

After about two days of reasonable quiet, I E-mailed Dennis Stillings, a friend in Hawaii, and told him I wanted work, had a few skills and some enthusiasm, and was still pretty cute. It was time for me to grow something, to put into practice all that I had been teaching and writing about. I have no idea why I chose to write this odd little résumé to Dennis and no one else, but I did. Maybe because I was on-line in the middle of the night, as usual, when an E-mail from Dennis whipped itself into my mailbox. Dennis is a biker turned archivist and knows more about the peculiar, the occult, and odd medical inventions than anyone I know.

Within a few days I was invited to go to the Big Island, and appointments were set up with many people at North Hawaiian Community Hospital and the Five Mountain Center. I had a lunch engagement with Earl Bakken, the inventor of the pacemaker, who has taken it as his personal responsibility to advance and sustain Hawaii's ancient reputation as the healing island.

North Hawaii Community Hospital was built in Waimea four years ago and is already known worldwide for its architecture and vision for health care. In the kitchen the cooks pray over the food, the nurses do healing touch, and plants suggested by "Papa" Henry Auwae, a kahuna who specialized in nutrition and botany, are around the door. By March a functional magnetic resonance imaging (fMRI) machine will be up and running, and I suppose this is what intrigues me most. There is no conceivable reason why an island that small would have such a state-of-the-art piece of equipment, but it does. And its acquisition was approved by the state of Hawaii only on the condition that it be used for research purposes at least eight hours a week.

Earl Bakken gave the hospital a grant for prayer studies, and the design and initiation of these is to be my first task. Since I've been receiving world-record-breaking amounts of prayer this past year, I've done some serious thinking about it. My research methodology skills will be challenged: the island has too small a population to permit large, randomized studies that would be statistically significant. But it does have the fMRI, which can detect minute and dynamic changes in physiology and be used, as could no other instrument, to track the biological effects of prayer, praying, imagery, or meditation. I find this terribly exciting, because if a positive correlation can be established, such a finding would shatter the barrier that has kept prayer out of medicine for so long.

Dr. Sam, the hospital's chaplain, had been with Mother Teresa in India for many years. He said, "Jeanne, this is a divine appointment for you. Please come." I knew that it was and that even if the work had been in Waco, Texas, I would feel compelled to go.

When I was asked what else I wanted to do there, I replied, "I want to develop a comprehensive center for the treatment of cancer patients." I had in mind what I had looked for all over the world but could not find: a place that focuses on health and the quality of life, uses a broad spectrum of treatments, and honors soul work. My ideal would be a place of aftercare and not necessarily primary treatment, a place where people who are essentially healthy could go to become healthier. I have committed to having this center designed within a year. It will be a pleasure. The island already has its own healing spirits of land and place, and with their cooperation, the center will be triumphant.

Last week the shamanic healing work that had begun with Michael Harner in September after the Grim Reaper diagnosis also came full circle. Michael and Sandy were on vacation at Kona Village the same time I was this year. Michael had spoken earlier about Lanakila Brandt, a kahuna pule (a medicine person who uses prayer and spirit for healing) who had worked with Michael several years ago. I asked Michael to help me visit the kahuna if he could, and an appointment was arranged for six days before I was to leave the island.

Lanakela visited with Michael, Sandy, and me and brought us the traditional awa, or kava-kava, tea. I knew he was watching me carefully, deciding whether we should work together. I tried to say and do the appropriate things but didn't really know what they were, except to honor his wisdom and be respectful. He is one of the few left in the islands who remembers the ancient teachings and one of the very few who focuses on prayer and spirituality. He is seventy-eight years old, quite fragile now, and has clear blue eyes. I must have passed his scrutiny. He and I had periodic waves of "chicken flesh," which demonstrated the active presence of the spirits.

Every day for five days, either Judy or Mo would accompany me to Lanakila's home, a two-hour round-trip drive. He would greet us in his yellow ceremonial robes and headband, and we sipped a cup of awa. Then my friend would wait outside, praying, and Lanakela would beckon me into a room that had been purified with water from the sea, sprinkled with ti leaves. The first day we each placed a ti-leaf lei around the god on the altar and blessed each other. Then, that day and every day thereafter, I lay down on a white bed, and Lanakela called in his ancestors' spirits and all the gods and goddesses of the pantheon.

He sang prayers over me for two hours each day—prayers of protection, healing, and power. He, I, and the altar were enveloped in a holy circle, as he seemed to be negotiating, talking, and listening to the spirits about my eye. I have never heard such beautiful sounds. He sang at first in English, elegant translations of his own making, and then eventually in Hawaiian only. He reminded me that I was a daughter of Pele, the fire goddess, and I forgave myself for my own intensity. My *mana* (life force) was strong, he, the gods and goddesses, and the ancestors assured me, and I would lead a rich and full life.

On our second day I appeared in the morning but could not settle down enough to take in the songs. I was wired, and Lanakila looked tired and weak. He assured me again and again that it was not my fault, that he simply was unable to communicate with the spirits, and would I come back that afternoon? Of course, I would. When I returned, was waiting for me with a book bound in bark cloth, with the translations of the songs and prayers. He said, "I know this will work better for you if I tell you what is going on." Then he continued, "I'm getting old, and very ready to join my mama and daddy. It is time for me to teach what I know so that it is not lost forever."

Not coincidentally, I suppose, on the third day I detected flashes of light on my retina—for the first time in more than a year. I do not know what this means except that my eye is more than half alive.

I asked permission to call my ancestors into the room as well as the spirits of my children, who needed healing. There was no question that the room was full of spirits, and what I felt was pure love. I surrendered and allowed myself to be carried wherever they needed me. During our last time together, I must have been very far away. Lanakila said one must not be brought back suddenly, but carefully and gently. He gradually awoke me with the sweetest sounds of an unfamiliar song: "Aloha, Jeanne. Aloha, aloha, Jeanne."

"Aloha."

I have been sung home. The spirits have more work for me to do.

Resources

A resource section in a book of this nature is rather unusual, I realize. However, as my adventure unfolded in both the traditional and alternative medical arenas, many people asked me about the individuals and places that I've found helpful. So below I've listed as many references as seemed reasonable, including contact information and Web sites whenever possible. This isn't a global endorsement but a statement of who and what was helpful in my particular experience.

BOOKS AND RECORDINGS

Achterberg, Jeanne. *Imagery in Healing: Shamanism and Modern Medicine.* Boston: Shambhala Publications, 1985.

———. *Woman as Healer.* Boston: Shambhala Publications, 1994.

———, Barbara Dossey, and Leslie Kolkmeier. *Rituals of Healing: Using Imagery for Health and Wellness.* New York: Bantam, 1994.

———, and G. Frank Lawlis. *Bridges of the Bodymind: Behavioral Approaches to Health Care.* Champaign, Ill.: Institute for Personality and Ability Testing, 1980.

Arrien, Angeles. *The Four-Fold Way: Walking the Paths of the Warrior, Teacher, Healer, and Visionary.* New York: HarperCollins, 1992.

———. *The Tarot Handbook: Principal Applications of Ancient Visual Symbols.* New York: Putnam, 1992.

———. *Signs of Life: The Five Universal Shapes and How to Use Them.* New York: Penguin/Putnam, 1998.

———. *The Nine Muses: A Mythological Path to Creativity.* New York: Putnam, 2000.

Bolen, Jean Shinoda. *Close to the Bone: Life-Threatening Illness and the Search for Meaning*. New York: Touchstone Books, 1998.

Broyard, Anatole. *Intoxicated by My Illness and Other Writings on Life and Death*. New York: Clarkson Potter, 1992.

Campbell, Don G. *The Mozart Effect: Tapping the Power of Music to Heal the Body, Strengthen the Mind, and Unlock the Creative Spirit*. New York: Avon Books, 1997.

———. *The Mozart Effect: Tapping the Power of Music to Heal the Body, Strengthen the Mind, and Unlock the Creative Spirit*. (audio cassettes) Brilliance Corp., 1997.

Dossey, Barbara. *Florence Nightingale: Mystic, Visionary, Healer*. New York: Springhouse, 2000.

———, Lynn Keegan, and Cathie Guzzetta. *Holistic Nursing: A Handbook for Practice*. Gaithersburg, Md.: Aspen Publishers, 2000.

Dossey, Larry, M.D. *Healing Words: The Power of Prayer and the Practice of Medicine*. San Francisco: HarperSanFrancisco, 1993.

———. *Be Careful What You Pray For . . . You Just Might Get It*. San Francisco: HarperSanFrancisco, 1997.

———. *Reinventing Medicine: Beyond Mind-Body to a New Era of Healing*. San Francisco: HarperSanFrancisco, 1999.

Gass, Robert, and Kathleen A. Brehony. *Chanting: Discovering Spirit in Sound*. New York: Broadway Books, 1999.

———. *Chant: Spirit in Sound*. (compact disc) Spring Hill, 2000.

Gordon, James S. *Manifesto for a New Medicine: Your Guide to Healing Partnerships and the Wise Use of Alternative Therapies*. Cambridge, Mass.: Perseus Publishing, 1997.

Harner, Michael J. *The Way of the Shaman*. San Francisco: HarperSanFrancisco, 1990.

Houston, Jean. *A Mythic Life: Learning to Live Our Greater Story*. San Francisco: HarperSanFrancisco, 1996.

———. *The Possible Human: A Course in Enhancing Your Physical, Mental, and Creative Abilities*. New York: J. P. Tarcher/Putnam, 1997.

———. *The Search for the Beloved: Journeys in Mythology and Sacred Psychology*. New York: J. P. Tarcher/Putnam, 1997.

———. *Jump Time: Shaping Your Future in a World of Radical Change*. New York: J. P. Tarcher/Putnam, 2000.

Hulme, Keri. *The Bone People*. New York: Penguin, 1986.

Ingerman, Sandra. *Soul Retrieval: Mending the Fragmented Self*. San Francisco: HarperSanFrancisco, 1991.

Lawson, Lee. *Visitations from the Afterlife: True Stories of Love and Healing*. New York: HarperCollins, 2000.

LeShan, Lawrence. *The Medium, the Mystic, and the Physicist: Toward a General Theory of the Paranormal*. New York: Viking Penguin, 1974.

———. *Cancer as a Turning Point: A Handbook for People with Cancer, Their Families, and Health Professionals*. New York: Dutton Signet, 1994.

O'Regan, Brendan, and Caryle Hirshberg. *Spontaneous Remission: An Annotated Bibliography*. Petaluma, Calif.: Institute of Noetic Sciences, 1995.

Shealy, C. Norman. *Miracles Do Happen: A Physician's Experience with Alternative Medicine*. New York: Element Books, 1995.

———. *Sacred Healing: The Curing Power of Energy and Spirituality*. New York: Element Books, 1999.

Simmons, Marc. *Witchcraft in the Southwest: Spanish and Indian Supernaturalism on the Rio Grande*. Lincoln, Nebr.: University of Nebraska Press, 1980.

Simonton, O. Carl., M.D., and Reid Henson with Brenda Hampton. *The Healing Journey*. New York: Bantam, 1994.

———, Stephanie Matthews-Simonton, and James L. Creighton. *Getting Well Again*. New York: Bantam Doubleday Dell, 1980.

PERIODICALS AND OTHER PUBLICATIONS

Alternative Therapies in Health and Medicine   A peer-reviewed journal that explores the use of alternative therapies in preventing and treating disease and promoting health (www.alternative-therapies.com).

The Cancer Chronicles   A newsletter published by Ralph Moss from 1989–1998; the archives of *The Cancer Chronicles* can be searched at www.ralphmoss.com.

The Moss Reports   Detailed reports on a wide variety of cancer types and situations (available through www.ralphmoss.com or www.cancerdecisions.com).

Sacred Space   A scholarly journal on spirituality and health care, edited by Steve Wright (for more information visit www.sacredspace.org.uk).

WEB SITES AND ORGANIZATIONS

Association of On-Line Cancer Resources
www.acor.org
This Web site sponsors mailing lists on cancer treatment and provides links to support groups, articles by cancer survivors, and access to CancerNet.

Lanakela Brandt
www.haleola.com/1999/Mana%20copy/Huna.html

Brandt is a kahuna pule, a Hawaiian medicine man, and an experienced practitioner of the native Hawaiian healing rite of la'au kahea, *the rite he performed on me in the book.*

Jean Shinoda Bolen, M.D.
www.jeanshinodabolen.com

A Jungian analyst, writer, teacher, and leader in the women's empowerment movement, Jean has a special interest in the psychological and spiritual dimensions of cancer and other serious illnesses.

Center for Mind-Body Medicine
5225 Connecticut Ave. NW, Suite 414
Washington, DC 20015
(202) 966-7338
www.cmbm.org

Directed by James Gordon, M.D., the Center for Mind-Body Medicine is dedicated to improving the practice of medicine through developing new models of care that incorporate the mental, emotional, and spiritual dimensions of health and illness.

David Cumes, M.D.
Inward Bound Healing Adventure
1114 Del Mar
Santa Barbara, CA 93109
(805) 564-2341

Inward Bound Healing Adventures takes people into remote wilderness areas and to ritual healers, offering participants an opportunity to connect with the healing power of nature as well as the healing practices of indigenous peoples.

Barbara Dossey, R.N.
www.dosseydossey.com/barbara

Barbara Dossey is the director of Holistic Nursing Consultants and a noted writer and teacher on holistic health.

Larry Dossey, M.D.
www.dosseydossey.com/larry

Larry Dossey is an influential thinker and writer on of the role of the mind in health and the role of spirituality in healthcare.

Esalen Institute
Highway 1
Big Sur, CA 93920
(831) 667-3000
www.esalen.org
Esalen is a much-loved alternative education center offering workshops that incorporate philosophy, psychology, and spirituality.

Five Mountain Medical Community
P.O. Box 7079
Kamuela, HI 96743-7079
(808) 885-9227
www.fivemtn.org
This is a regional community development initiative that is shaping a unique model of health and healing.

Foundation for Shamanic Studies
P.O. Box 1939
Mill Valley, CA 94942
(415) 380-8282
www.shamanism.org
This is the educational organization founded by Michael Harner, pioneering anthropologist and shaman.

The Gerson Institute
P.O. Box 430
Bonita, CA 91908
www.gerson-research.org
This organization studies the impact of diet and nutrition on cancer and other diseases and publishes educational materials and newsletters.

Nicholas J. Gonzalez, M.D.
www.dr-gonzalez.com
Gonzalez is a leading researcher studying the role of nutrition in the treatment of cancer and other degenerative diseases.

Sandra Ingerman
www.shamanism.org/fssinfo/singerbio.html
Sandra Ingerman is the leading practitioner of soul retrieval.

Institute of Health and Healing
PO. Box 7999
California Pacific Medical Center
San Francisco, CA 94120

IHH pioneered efforts in offering complementary and alternative medical care and sponsors educational and research programs.

Institute of Noetic Sciences
101 San Antonio Rd.
Petaluma, CA 94952
(707) 775-3500
www.noetic.org

IONS is dedicated to scientific research of consciousness and the human potential.

Lawrence LeShan
www.cancerasaturningpoint.org

Larry LeShan is considered by many to be the father of mind-body medicine.

Ralph Moss, Ph.D.
www.ralphmoss.com

Moss is an acclaimed science writer and medical investigator specializing in cancer.

National Center for Complementary and Alternative Medicine (NCCAM)
NCCAM Clearinghouse
P.O. Box 8218
Silver Spring, MD 20907-8218
(888) 644-6226 (toll-free)
nccam.nih.gov/nccam

This is the division of the National Institutes of Health that researches complementary and alternative therapies.

The National Foundation for Alternative Medicine
1629 K Street N.W., Suite 402
Washington, D.C. 20006
(202) 463-4900
www.nfam.org

NFAM was founded by Berkley Bedell, a former U.S. Congressman and cancer survivor. The foundation researches and publicizes information about

alternative and complementary treatments for cancer and other diseases and
makes its findings available to the public free of charge.

North Hawaii Community Hospital
67-1125 Mamalahoa Hwy.
Kamuela, HI 96743
(808) 885-4444
planet-hawaii.com/nhch
This hospital is a prototype for the integration of modern medicine and
alternative and complementary therapies.

Mark Rennecker, M.D.
(415) 681-6044
An excellent medical detective who will research diagnoses and treatment
options and is familiar with many systems of healing.

The Sacred Space Foundation
Ravenscroft
Renwick, Cumbria CA10 1JL
England
www.sacredspace.org.uk
Headed by Steve Wright and Jean Sayre-Adams, this organization is dedicated
to caring for caregivers, especially professionals, who have become exhausted and
burned out in their work.

Saybrook Graduate School
450 Pacific, Third Floor
San Francisco, CA 94133
(800) 825-4480 (toll-free)
www.saybrook.edu
Saybrook offers long-distance graduate programs in psychology, human science,
and organizational systems inquiry.

Bernie Siegel, M.D.
c/o Exceptional Cancer Patients
1302 Chapel Street
New Haven, CT 06511
(203) 865-8392
Dr. Siegel is an internationally known pioneer in cancer mind/body therapy.

Simonton Cancer Center
P.O. Box 890
Pacific Palisades, CA 90272
(800) 459-3424 (toll-free)
www.simontoncenter.com

The Simonton Cancer Center offers retreat programs for cancer patients based on Simonton's ground-breaking research into the psychological dimensions of cancer.